INTRODUCTION TO QUANTITATIVE RESEARCH METHODS

INTRODUCTION TO QUANTITATIVE RESEARCH METHODS

AN INVESTIGATIVE APPROACH

MARK BALNAVES and
PETER CAPUTI

SAGE Publications
London • Thousand Oaks • New Delhi

SAGE Publications Ltd
6 Bonhill Street
London EC2A 4PU

SAGE Publications Inc
2455 Teller Road
Thousand Oaks, California 91320

SAGE Publications India Pvt Ltd
32, M-Block Market
Greater Kailash-I
New Delhi 110 048

British Library Cataloguing in Publication data

A catalogue record for this book is
available from the British Library

ISBN 0-7619-6803-2
ISBN 0-7619-6804-0 (pbk)

Library of Congress catalog record available

Typeset by Keyword Publishing Services Limited, UK
Printed in Great Britain by The Cromwell Press Ltd,
Trowbridge, Wiltshire

Contents

CONTENTS

Tables

Figures

Acknowledgements

A special thanks to:

Gary Bouma and David DeVaus

Mark Busani, Nick Castle and Monica Vecchiotti for their help with the multimedia courseware.

Maurice Dunlevy, for contributions on journalism, and Harry Oxley, for contributions on causal diagramming.

Patrick Rawstorne for use of his PhD dataset Predicting and Explaining the use of Information Technology with Value Expectancy Models of Behaviour in Contexts of Mandatory Use.

Erika Pearson – it's hard to find good help nowadays.

Tony Bennett, Mike Emmison and John Frow for use of their dataset from The Australian Everyday Consumption project.

SPSS illustrations have been reprinted by SPSS copyright permission. Excel illustrations have been reprinted by Excel copyright permission.

The Apple University Consortium and PCTech for their equipment and software support.

The Australian National Library for assistance with access to *The Strand*, from which the original Paget sketches of Sherlock Holmes were reproduced for this book.

Alec McHoul, Mike Innes, Joyce and Michele Balnaves, Wendy Parkins and James Donald, who provided valuable insights into detection.

John and Paul Balnaves on questions of Shakespeare and logic.

Michele, Mary-Claire, Gerard, Elayne, James, and Jack.

Douglas Adams – the bottle of red has been sent.

The authors of detective fiction.

Permissions

The authors and publishers wish to thank the following for their permission to use copyright material:

Tables 6.16 and 6.17. Copyright © 1993. Canadian Psychological Association. Reprinted with permission.

Page 12, extract from *The Strange Crime of John Boulnois* by G.K. Chesterton. Used by permission of A.P. Watt on behalf of The Royal Literary Fund.

Page 14, extract from *Dirk Gently's Holistic Detective Agency* by Douglas Adams. Used by permission of Douglas Adams. Copyright © 1987. Heinemann.

Figure 2.1. From *Evaluating Social Science Research*, second edition, by Paul C. Stern and Linda Kalof. Copyright © 1979, 1996. Oxford University Press, Inc. Used by permission of Oxford University Press.

Table 2.2. Used by permission of Gary Bouma. Copyright © 1993. *The Research Process*. Oxford University Press.

Page 38, extract from *The Blue Cross* by G.K. Chesterton. Used by permission of A.P. Watt on behalf of The Royal Literary Fund.

Figure 4.3. Used by permission of David DeVaus. Copyright © 1990. *Surveys in Social Research*. Allen and Unwin.

Table 4.7. From *Research Methods in Social Relations*, sixth edition, by Charles M. Judd, Eliot R. Smith and Louise H. Kidder. Copyright © 1991, Holt, Rinehart and Winston. Reproduced by permission of the publishers.

Every effort has been made to trace all copyright holders, but if any have been overlooked, or if any additional information can be given, the publishers will be pleased to make the necessary amendments at the first opportunity.

1

Order at All Points

Counting and accounting

A man is driving through the bush one day and has to stop while a farmer takes his sheep across the road. There are quite a lot of sheep, so it takes a fair while. When they've all passed by, the man goes up to the farmer and asks, 'If I can tell you how many sheep you have, to within one either way, can I have one of them?' The farmer replies, 'Course you can. You'll never get it right.' The man says, 'You have six thousand four hundred and twenty two.' 'Well blow me down,' replies the farmer – or words to that effect. 'In fact I have six thousand four hundred and twenty one. I counted them this morning.' So the man walks back to the car with his prize.

'Wait on,' cries the farmer. 'If I can tell you what your job is, can I have her back?' 'Sure,' says the man, 'You'll never guess.' 'Well,' says the farmer, 'I figure you'd be a statistician with the Australian Bureau of Statistics.' 'Well I'll be …!' the man replies, 'Exactly right. How on earth did you know that?'

The farmer comes back: 'Put me dog down and I'll tell you.'

Traditional Australian Bush Yarn

THE Ql-Qt CONTINUUM[1]

Like many in the humanities and social sciences, I was trained to be (at the least) sceptical about statistical methods and (at most) downright hostile towards them. In sceptical mode, I was exhorted to use statistics *not* in the way a drunk uses a lamppost: for support rather than illumination. In hostile mode, the word was that statistics was for 'positivists' (a very unfair characterization, as it turns out, of positivism). What all of this well-meaning and humanistic advice ignored was the sheer fact that our social and cultural worlds, today, are massively subject to statistical accounts (see Hacking, 1982). Whenever we turn on the TV news or open a newspaper, the world is now routinely accounted for in terms of the numbers it generates: from world population statistics right down to chewing gum markets. In this respect, it's not quite as if numbers were on one side of the coin and 'lived cultures' on the other. Rather, the technologies of numbering have become just one (though, in some disciplines, a dominant one) of the many practices that make up the cultures of modernity. In this brief introduction, then, I want to think through the supposed distinction (binary, even) between the quantitative (Qt) and the qualitative (Ql) and to show that the seal between the two is by no means as watertight as it is often assumed to be.

My first realization of an elision between Qt and Ql came to me when, out of sheer impecuniousness, I went to work for the Survey Research Centre at the Australian National University (ANU) in the mid-1970s. Prior to this way of supplementing my meagre PhD scholarship, my only encounter with statistics had been the compulsory undergraduate methods course in sociology, taught, as it happened, by a died-in-the-wool symbolic interactionist, a Ql-man if ever there was one! Said lecturer was, then, very happy for me to complete my statistics assignments by having a friend who was a physics student crunch the exercises on the university's one mainframe computer by submitting bundles of punchcards. Not, then, exactly the best of trainings or qualifications, I admit. But working late at ANU, designing and administering the Australian Capital Territory (ACT) population surveys, I came to see what a symbolic and interactional process Qt work could be in practice. One of our clients at the time was the local Family Planning organization. It wanted to know which forms of contraception were most in use in the Capital Territory. The only problem with this was that the official sampling procedures required interviewers to jointly interview two members of each household selected (using lot numbers) on a rotational basis: oldest and third oldest in odd-numbered lots, and second oldest and fourth oldest in even-numbered lots. This meant, in effect, that a fair proportion of interviews involved parents and their older children – not exactly the best interactional setting to ask people about their contraceptive practices. The problem was both, and equally, statistical and 'cultural.' Qt and Ql could not be a simple binary. And, oh yes, the wonderful 'solution' we developed was to draw up a card with each kind of contraception numbered. Respondents were then shown the card and would say such things as 'Well, I tried the number seven but it didn't work for me, so now I prefer the twenty six.'

The same realization came back to me during a more recent research project (Mickler and McHoul, 1998). In this project, we collected over 600 newspaper articles on Aborigines, youth and crime over a 12-month period in the early 1990s in order to see whether there had been, as some suspected at the time, a media-generated 'crime wave.' We had a neutral reader/research-assistant type the articles into a relational database program (QSR NUD·IST) and, at the same time, code the articles for such things as 'source' (the origin of the reported events), 'participants' (the categories of persons reported on in each article) and how the reader thought the article was treating such 'participants' (in positive, negative or neutral moral terms). What we hoped to get out of this was a strongly Ql argument based on a discursive analysis of the news articles and their 'readings.' However, before long, we found that working with over 600 texts would not allow us to do this. The data in question were simply too numerous. And anyway, NUD·IST was starting to generate matrices of such things as 'Date of publication' × 'Article source' and 'Newspaper' × 'Participants.' Each cell of the matrix listed the relevant articles by their unique NUD·IST document number. There was no way we could work with this

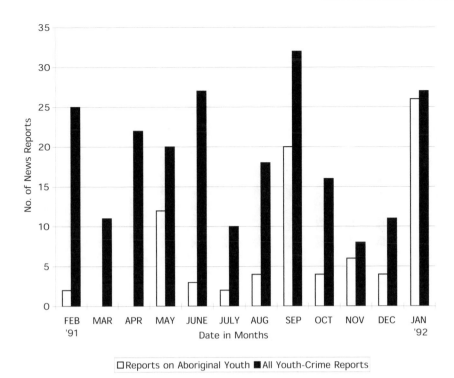

CHART 1.1   *Reports on Aboriginal youth and all youth-crime reports, Feb. 1991 to Jan. 1992*

kind of output in a purely Ql mode. We had to show our findings graphically. This meant a lot of arduous work, transferring the totals of each cell into an Excel spreadsheet and then having Excel generate graphs and bar charts. (This was in NUD·IST version 3: the day we finished our gruelling transcription work, NUD·IST 4 was released, including new software that automatically converts such findings into popular spreadsheet and stats programs.) At that point we were able to generate 'findings' such as those in Chart 1.1.

This was very useful to us because it showed us a picture of the year's news in terms of just when the WA press was reporting youth crimes, and the months during which young Aboriginal people were the 'participants' in those reports. However, while this could show us the media angle, it could not tell us whether or not the 'peaks' of youth crime reportage (and we were particularly interested in the September peak because it followed the infamous Rally for Justice outside Parliament House in the August) corresponded to 'actual' crime rates. If we were going to find a 'media wave,' we would have to overlay crime stats on to our bar chart. We eventually tracked these down at the University of Western Australia Crime Research Centre whose staff kindly gave us their raw figures for the 12-month period in question. Accordingly we could then generate more conclusive findings about the supposed 'wave' – see Chart 1.2.

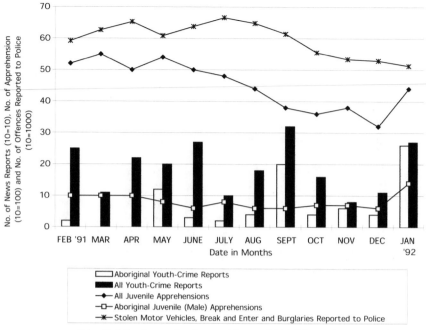

(Crime Statistics Sources: Broadhurst and Ferrante (1995: 87); Broadhurst and Loh (1995: 72))

CHART 1.2   *News reports on Aboriginal youth-crime and all youth-crime with actual crime data,*
Feb. 1991 to Jan. 1992

So we now had something like a 'media wave.' That is, as the reportage of youth crime peaked in September there was a corresponding decline in 'actual' crimes as measured by apprehensions and reports to the police.

Again, we could only see this graphically – though later we resorted to a more Ql discussion of how, in terms of routine media practices, the 'wave' could have been generated. That is, we wanted to show, from a close reading of the reports (in line with well-known facts about the news profession (Ericson et al., 1987, 1989, 1991)) that the statistically visible 'wave' was not so much a conscious conspiracy as a routine phenomenon in the field of 'bad news as usual.' As so frequently, the raw stats were open to more than one interpretation and only one of these was that the media were 'deliberately' causing the appearance of a crime wave with possibly suspect and populist motives.

Working on this project, then, brought me to the realization that there is in fact a continuum between hypothetically 'pure' Qt and Ql analysis. The two, that is, never actually exist, empirically, in their pure states. Qt work is part of the 'culture' at large and Ql work is never strictly free of numbers. So why then is there an effective stand-off between professionals in the two methodological fields? Why do some Qt workers insist on accepted sampling procedures and statistical reliability while some Ql workers argue that very small fragments of cultural 'data' (a poem, a few turns at talk, an advertisement, and so on) can generate just as fruitful findings? In order to begin to answer this question, we can turn to a rather extreme case of an anti-Qt argument. The one I have in mind was mounted some years ago by another major influence on my own methodological preferences: Harvey Sacks.

CULTURE AND THE RELIABILITY OF 'DATA'[2]

Just as in physics, natural phenomena must be massively sampled before an argument about their properties can be mounted, so, in some branches of the social sciences, cases must be sufficiently large in number before generalizations can be acceptable to the professional community. The parallel is both noble and mistaken, according to several social theorists of (roughly) a phenomenological persuasion. Alfred Schütz, many years ago, and in works that are almost unknown to Qt types today, put this argument very simply (Schütz, 1962: 34-47). He noticed that natural scientists deal with objects of the *first* order of interpretation: that is, the objects that the natural scientist has before her have not been interpreted until she herself shows up on the scene. Atoms, planets and cyclones do not interpret themselves. However, as soon as we come to deal with human individuals or populations, we're in a different situation entirely. These 'objects of knowledge' *have* interpreted themselves before the social scientist comes on the scene. They are therefore 'objects' of the *second* order of interpretation. They come pre-interpreted – and so the job of anyone working in the human sciences is to interpret the interpretations that people have already made of their lives (individually) and their cultures (collectively). Where human beings are concerned (as opposed to rats or atoms), the investigator is always investigating 'second order' matters. It is a fundamental category mistake, then, to treat humanly produced data as 'natural' data – though, as we will see shortly, this logical error need not preclude Qt analysis altogether: I am simply taking this argument as one of the most cogent to date on the underlying 'philosophy' of much Qt thinking.

Sacks's important intervention into this debate – possibly via his association with Garfinkel (1967) who was, in turn, majorly influenced by Schütz – is to argue for a unique position for cultural 'data.' Not only, he ventures, is culture distinct from nature, it also has unique orderly properties. That is: in coming to analyse human cultures, one must take into account that they display 'order at all points.' The argument is complex and students would do best to consult the original (1995: 484). However, Schegloff (who introduces both volumes) puts the matter succinctly. Accordingly, I quote at length:

> Considerations of enculturation and 'language acquisition' provide an especially provocative focus for a matter which Sacks raises ... as a methodological point.

> Taking up the relevance of sampling, Sacks points out that it depends on the sort of order one takes it that the social world exhibits. An alternative to the possibility that order manifests itself at an aggregate level and is statistical in character is what he terms the 'order at all points' view.... This view, rather like the 'holographic' model of information distribution, understands order not to be present only at aggregate levels and therefore subject to an overall differential distribution, but to be present in detail on a case by case, environment by environment basis. A culture is not then to be found only by aggregating all of its venues; it is substantially present in each of its venues. (Schegloff in Sacks 1995: xlvi)

As with holographs, a culture must display its inherent order, no matter how *much* or *little* of it we happen to examine or 'sample.' (And, as we will see shortly, this importantly applies as much to the 'much' as it does to the 'little.') Even if 99 per cent of a holographic image is destroyed, the remaining 1 per cent contains all of the information contained in the original whole (Roe, 1998). In this respect, when we are dealing with social and cultural phenomena (such as 'mental illness' or 'suicide,' for example), the question of whether we have sufficient cases for the 'data' to be 'reliable' may not arise. The order we are seeking, as social scientists or cultural analysts, according to Sacks, is not available as a form of statistical aggregation; rather it must be inherently present in whatever materials happen to be at hand – for example just a few turns in a conversation. And, in fact, Sacks directly uses his 'order at all points' (or 'in all venues') model to criticize Qt research. His argument here is particularly directed at sociology and survey research, but it applies equally well to the other social sciences:

> ... you might find that the fact of 'order at all points' could be used to explain fairly strange facts; things like the following. For one, certain kinds of researches – for example, let's say, taking very conventional sociology, survey research – would use the fact that it gets orderly results to indicate that it must be doing something decent. Now everybody knows – that is, everybody who has ever done such work, or studied it – that it's almost universally extremely bad; that almost never can whatever the constraints are that ought to be used under their own formulation to decide that they have something, be used. There are, for example, all kinds of constraints on proper statistical procedures which are never satisfied, and *none the less they get order*. (1995: 484, my emphasis)

The argument here is important: the reason why Qt procedures arrive at orderly outcomes may *not* be because of the 'reliability' of either the sample or the statistical techniques deployed on that sample. Rather, the order that arises would be, for Sacks, an effect of the fact that, wherever a culture is tapped into, and however frequently or infrequently it is sampled, it will display its *inherent* order. If this is the case – and I have yet to see a social theory that directly defends an aggregationist model against the idea of 'order at all points' – then statistically reliable results may well be nothing more than a case of something intrinsically non-statistical showing through (and despite) the sampling techniques employed in any given case. The consequences of such a 'paradigm shift' are potentially massive for social scientific thinking – not least because they might change our thinking away from what Wittgenstein (1958b: 18) called our 'craving for generality' and/ or 'the contemptuous attitude towards the particular case' (cf. Turner, 1974: 213).

However, none of this means that Qt work is without value.[3] On the contrary, as we have seen in our first section of this introduction, statistical representations are sometimes inevitable: and in the above case, the reason for this had to do with the necessarily longitudinal nature of the 'media wave' hypothesis. If this is so – and because Ql and Qt exist on a continuum and not as strict alternatives – then even the most Ql-oriented researchers will occasionally find themselves needing to use statistical models and their ensuing graphic representations. If the 'continuum' argument holds up (and I think it does, at least from experience), then how can this live in the same world as the 'order at all points' argument?

Sacks himself gives us the answer when he writes that, even when we do proceed statistically, and even in its crudest form (the survey), we will find the same cultural order as when we do not! 'None the less they get order' is precisely what he tells us. That is, if cultural 'data' is intrinsically data of the second order, any statistical analysis of it *cannot help but preserve* that aspect of it. The 'philosophy' of treating social and cultural phenomena as if they were natural phenomena may well be a philosophical error – associated (probably wrongly) with 'positivism.' But this does not mean that the *methods* that flow from that error can somehow delete the orderly cultural properties of the former kind of phenomenon. In fact, Sacks himself tells us that they *could* not even if they wanted to.

This then sets the tone – or more precisely, the 'analytic mentality' (Schenkein, 1978) – for the following chapters of this book.[4] They introduce some central *social and cultural* uses of Qt methods and, at the same time, always remember the importance of the 'order at all points' that such uses must bring out. Or to put this another way: there is no logical reason why Qt methods can't be just as informed by a Sacksian view of cultural order as they can by starting 'positivistically' with physics envy. The result is, I think, the first textbook in the field to bring cultural responsiveness to statistical methods and, equally, statistical responsibility to cultural analysis.

Alec McHoul
Murdoch University

NOTES

1. This sub-title with apologies to *Star Trek TNG*. In many way, *Star Trek*'s Q is the *ultimate* detective. His case is nothing more or less than the human condition.

2. This section is based on parts of an article on Sacks, conversation analysis and psychology by Alec McHoul and Mark Rapley (2000). For a good general introduction to Sacks, see Silverman (1998).

3. For example, the foundational text of ethnomethodology, Garfinkel's *Studies in Ethnomethodology* (1967), extensively uses statistical and quasi-statistical representations to show 'experimental' results.

4. I write 'more precisely' with half an eye on the problem of what 'precision' could mean on the Ql–Qt continuum. To explain: the term 'analytic mentality' is from Jim Schenkein (1978). He writes: 'I am never entirely sure of what I mean by "analytic mentality", but then goes on to say: 'I have come to think of [our] shared practices [in conversation analysis] as ingredients in an "analytic mentality" since other more familiar terms fail to capture the spectrum of ingredients sketched here. Our particular grouping of shared dispositions is not exactly a "theory" or "method", nor is it merely a "point of view" or some kind of "philosophy". But whatever it is, the result is a research environment . . . and "analytic mentality" is fuzzy enough to embrace whatever comes up when a closer look at the environment is taken' (1978: 6). So this fuzzy formulation seems to be, paradoxically perhaps, a more *precise* description than terms like 'theory' and 'method'. This would be exactly my characterization of work that explicitly acknowledges and works along the Ql–Qt continuum. As Wittgenstein (1958a: #71) puts it: 'Is it . . . always an advantage to replace an indistinct picture by a sharp one? Isn't the indistinct one often exactly what we need?'

REFERENCES

Broadhurst, Roderic and Ferrante, Anna (1995) 'Trends in juvenile crime and justice, 1990–1992', in R. Harding (ed.) *Repeat Juvenile Offenders: The Failure of Selective Incapacitation in Western Australia*. Nedlands, WA: Crime Research Centre, University of Western Australia. pp. 79–95.

Broadhurst, Roderic and Loh, Nini Sui Nie (1995) 'Selective incapacitation and the phantom of deterrence', in R. Harding (ed.) *Repeat Juvenile Offenders: The Failure of Selective Incapacitation in Western Australia*. Nedlands, WA: Crime Research Centre, University of Western Australia. pp. 55–78.

Ericson, Richard, Baranek, Patricia and Chan, Janet (1987) *Visualizing Deviance: A Study of News Organization*. Toronto: University of Toronto Press.

Ericson, Richard, Baranek, Patricia and Chan, Janet (1989) *Negotiating Control: A Study of News Sources*. Stony Stratford: Open University Press.

Ericson, Richard, Baranek, Patricia and Chan, Janet (1991) *Representing Order: Crime, Law, and Justice in the News Media*. Buckingham: Open University Press.

Garfinkel, Harold (1967) *Studies in Ethnomethodology*. Englewood Cliffs: Prentice-Hall.

Hacking, Ian (1982) 'Biopower and the avalanche of printed numbers', *Humanities in Society*, 5 (3/4): pp. 279–95.

McHoul, Alec and Rapley, Mark (2000) 'Sacks and clinical psychology', *Clinical Psychology Forum*, 142 (August): pp. 5–12.

Mickler, Steve and McHoul, Alec (1998) 'Sourcing the wave: Crime reporting, Aboriginal youth and the WA Press, Feb 1991–Jan 1992', *Media International Australia incorporating Culture and Policy*, 86 (February): pp. 122–52.

Roe, Phil (1998) *Of Hologrammatology: The Politics of Virtual Writing.* Unpublished PhD thesis, Murdoch University.

Sacks, Harvey (1995) *Lectures on Conversation, Vol. 1.* Ed. G. Jefferson, intro. E.A. Schegloff. Oxford: Blackwell.

Schenkein, Jim (1978) 'Sketch of an analytic mentality for the study of conversational interaction', In J. Schenkein (ed.) *Studies in the Organization of Conversational Interaction.* New York: Academic Press. pp. 1–6.

Schütz, Alfred (1962) *Collected Papers Vol. 1: The Problem of Social Reality.* Ed. and intro. M. Natanson. The Hague: Martinus Nijhoff.

Silverman, David (1998) *Harvey Sacks: Social Science and Conversation Analysis.* Cambridge: Polity Press.

Turner, Roy (1974) 'Words, utterances and activities', in R. Turner (ed.) *Ethnomethodology: Selected Readings.* London: Penguin. pp. 197–215.

Wittgenstein, Ludwig (1958a) *Philosophical Investigations.* 2nd edn. Trans. G.E.M. Anscombe. Oxford: Blackwell.

Wittgenstein, Ludwig (1958b) *The Blue and Brown Books: Preliminary Studies for the 'Philosophical Investigations'.* Oxford: Blackwell.

2

Starting the Inquiry

'But what happened then?'

'I'll tell you what happened then,' said Fiennes with a grim emphasis.
'When we got back into that garden the first thing we saw was Traill, the lawyer; I can see him now with his black hat and black whiskers relieved against the perspective of the blue flowers stretching down to the summer-house, with the sunset and the strange outline of the Rock of Fortune in the distance. His face and figure were in shadow against the sunset; but I swear the white teeth were showing in his head and he was smiling.
'The moment Nox saw that man the dog dashed forward and stood in the middle of the path barking at him madly, murderously, volleying out curses that were almost verbal in their dreadful distinctness of hatred. And the man doubled up and fled along the path between the flowers.'

The Oracle of the Dog

Fiennes was a friend of Father Brown, G.K. Chesterton's famous priest-detective. Fiennes was recounting a story to Father Brown about the reaction of Nox, the dog, to a lawyer who represented Colonel Druce, a wealthy man who had only recently been murdered. The newspapers had reported that Druce had been murdered with a sharp knife in a garden with no outside entry. The witnesses saw no murderer and there was no knife. Fiennes thought that the dog's reaction to Traill the lawyer was a clear sign that the lawyer was the murderer.

Father Brown, however, interrogates his friend further and discovers that Colonel Druce changed his will and left his money to his daughter, rather than to his son Harry Druce, who owed money from gambling. Harry Druce committed suicide after his father's death. Father Brown also found out that the dog had tried to retrieve something from the ocean on a walk with Fiennes at the time of the murder and came back empty handed. Father Brown comes to the conclusion that Colonel Druce, who wore a white coat, was visible through a hedge that surrounded the garden. A man with a walking-stick-knife had seen Druce through the hedge and stabbed him. The man had then thrown the walking-stick-knife into the ocean. The dog tried to retrieve the walking stick, but to no avail because it sank. Harry Druce was the man who killed Colonel Druce. Harry killed himself when he realized that his murder was in vain and that his severe debts would not be resolved.

Fiennes is amazed that Father Brown can work out the crime from a distance. Father Brown replies, 'You asked how I could guess things a hundred miles away but honestly it's mostly to your credit, for you described people so well that I know the types.' Father Brown rejected Fiennes's interpretation of the dog's reaction to Traill and instead broadened the inquiry. 'I had a sort of guess,' said Father Brown, 'right at the beginning when you said that Druce wore a white coat.'

Father Brown was not a Columbo or a Hercule Poirot, who often as not started their investigations knowing who the crook was. Father Brown started his inquiries into mysterious unsolved crimes by collecting a wide range of accounts and observations, no matter how zany or far fetched those accounts and observations might superficially look. Father Brown did not assume that the context of a crime was obvious and that knowledge of that context came from looking at only a few clues. Father Brown carefully weighs up what he has found (what he thinks is a clue) and the logical consequences of what he has found (what he thinks must rationally follow).

In *The Strange Crime of John Boulnois* (Chesterton, 1987), Father Brown arrives at a scene where an American journalist has witnessed the death of Sir Claude Champion, dressed as Romeo and stabbed with a sword, saying with his last breath 'Boulnois ... with my own sword ... he threw it ...'. The journalist was on his way to interview John Boulnois, an 'Oxford man' who had recently published a review on Darwinian evolution. Father Brown interviews the wife of John Boulnois.

'Father Brown' she said.
'Mrs. Boulnois?' he replied gravely. Then he looked at her and immediately said: 'I see you know about Sir Claude.'
'How do you know I know?' she asked steadily. [*emphasis added*]
He did not answer the question, but asked another: 'Have you seen your husband?'
'My husband is at home,' she said. 'He has nothing to do with this.'
Again he did not answer; and the woman drew nearer to him, with a curiously intense expression on her face.
'Shall I tell you something more?' she said, with a rather fearful smile. 'I don't think he did it, and *you* don't either.'
Father Brown returned her gaze with a long, grave stare, and then nodded, yet more gravely.
'Father Brown,' said the lady, 'I am going to tell you all I know, but I want you to do me a favour first. Will you tell me *why* you haven't jumped to the conclusion of poor John's guilt, as all the rest have done? Don't mind what you say: I–I know about the gossip and the appearances that are against him.'
Father Brown looked honestly embarrassed and passed his hand across his forehead. 'Two very little things,' he said. 'At least one's very trivial and the other very vague. But such as they are, they don't fit in with Mr. Boulnois being the murderer.'
He turned his blank, round face up to the stars and continued absent mindedly: 'To take the vague idea first. I attach a good deal of importance to vague ideas. **All those things that 'aren't evidence' are what convince me.** [*emphasis added*] I think a moral impossibility the biggest of all impossibilities. I know your husband only slightly, but I think this crime of his, as generally conceived, something very like a moral impossibility. Please do not think I mean that Boulnois could not be so

wicked. Anybody can be wicked – as wicked as he chooses. We can direct our moral wills; but we can't generally change our instinctive tastes and ways of doing things. Boulnois might commit a murder, but not this murder. He would not snatch Romeo's sword from its romantic scabbard; or slay his foe on the sundial as on a kind of altar; or leave his body among the roses; or fling the sword away among the pines. If Boulnois killed anyone he'd do it quietly and heavily, as he'd do any other doubtful thing – take a tenth glass of port, or read a loose Greek poet. No, the romantic setting is not like Boulnois. It's more like Champion.'

'Ah!' she said, and looked at him with eyes like diamonds.

'And the trivial thing was this,' said Brown. 'There were fingerprints on that sword; fingerprints can be detected quite a time after they are made if they're on some polished surface like glass or steel. These were on a polished surface. They were half-way down the blade of the sword. Whose prints they were I have no earthly clue; but why should anybody hold a sword half-way down? It was a long sword, but length is an advantage in lunging at an enemy. At least, at most enemies. At all enemies except one.'

'Except one!' she repeated.

'There is only one enemy,' said Father Brown, 'whom it is easier to kill with a dagger than a sword.'

'I know,' said the woman. 'Oneself.'

There was a long silence, and then the priest said quietly but abruptly: 'Am I right, then? Did Sir Claude kill himself?'

'Yes,' she said, with a face like marble. 'I saw him do it.'

'He died,' said Father Brown, 'for love of you?'

An extraordinary expression flashed across her face, very different from pity, modesty, remorse, or anything her companion had expected: her voice became suddenly strong and full. 'I don't believe,' she said, 'he ever cared about me a rap. He hated my husband.'

'Why?' asked the other, and turned his round face from the sky to the lady.

'He hated my husband because . . . it is so strange I hardly know how to say it . . . because . . .'

'Yes?' said Brown patiently.

'Because my husband wouldn't hate him.'

Father Brown only nodded, and seemed still to be listening; he differed from most detectives in fact and fiction in a small point – he never pretended not to understand when he understood perfectly well.

Mrs. Boulnois drew near once more with the same contained glow of certainty. 'My husband,' she said, 'is a great man. Sir Claude Champion was not a great man: he was a celebrated and successful man. My husband has never been celebrated or successful; and it is the solemn truth that he has never dreamed of being so. He no more expected to be famous for thinking than for smoking cigars. On all that side he has a sort of splendid stupidity. He has never grown up. He still liked Champion exactly as he liked him at school; he admired him as he would admire a conjuring trick done at the dinner-table. But he couldn't be got to conceive the notion of *envying* Champion. *And Champion wanted to be envied.* He went mad and killed himself for that.'

(Used by permission)

Father Brown's detection style is summarized in his enigmatic comment 'All those things that "aren't evidence" are what convince me'. Father

Brown tries to avoid preconceived hypotheses and preconceived ideas about the relevance of the things that he observes. Father Brown works from 'inside out', carefully analysing all the events and clues (including witness accounts) and then drawing conclusions based on the evidence.

In many of the Father Brown stories, of course, there is something Father Brown knows that we do not know. We only find out at the end of the story how Father Brown reached his conclusions and why. The detective's knowledge and the reader's knowledge are not always the same during a story. For Father Brown and the reader, however, there are only a finite number of interpretations of accounts available to explain the crime mystery. Indeed, we would not want to read detective fiction if we thought that *any story* accounted for what had happened.

If Father Brown works from the 'inside out' in his collection and analysis of evidence, then Sherlock Holmes is perhaps the perfect example of the detective who works from the 'outside in'. Father Brown, like Holmes, always held that there is a rational explanation for all things. Father Brown, though, is seen as the inquisitive interviewer, collecting individual facts and then solving the crime. Sherlock Holmes, in contrast, argued that he could deduce the solution to the whole crime from only a few facts. Holmes always enjoyed demonstrating his 'powers of deduction' with Dr Watson. Dr Watson recounts this scene from *A Scandal in Bohemia*.

One night – it was on the twentieth of March, 1888—I was returning from a journey to a patient (for I had now returned to civil practice), when my way led me through Baker Street. As I passed the well-remembered door, which must always be associated in my mind with my wooing, and with the dark incidents of *The Study in Scarlet*, I was seized with a keen desire to see Holmes again, and to know how he was employing his extraordinary powers. His rooms were brilliantly lit, and, even as I looked up, I saw his tall, spare figure pass twice in a dark silhouette against the blind. He was pacing the room swiftly, eagerly, with his head sunk upon his chest and his hands clasped behind him. To me, who knew his every mood and habit, his attitude and manner told their own story. He was at work again. He had risen out of his drug-created dreams and was hot upon the scent of some new problem. I rang the bell and was shown up to the chamber which had formerly been in part my own.

His manner was not effusive. It seldom was; but he was glad, I think, to see me. With hardly a word spoken, but with a kindly eye, he waved me to an armchair, threw across his case of cigars, and indicated a spirit case and a gasogene in the corner. Then he stood before the fire and looked me over in his singular introspective fashion.

'Wedlock suits you,' he remarked. 'I think, Watson, that you have put on seven and a half pounds since I saw you.'

'Seven!' I answered.

'Indeed, I should have thought a little more. Just a trifle more, I fancy, Watson. And in practice again, I observe. You did not tell me that you intended to go into harness.'

'Then, how do you know?'

'I see it, I deduce it. [*emphasis added*] How do I know that you have been getting yourself very wet lately, and that you have a most clumsy and careless servant girl?'

'My dear Holmes,' said I, 'this is too much. You would certainly have been burned, had you lived a few centuries ago. It is true that I had a country walk on Thursday and came home in a dreadful mess, but as I have changed my clothes I can't imagine how you deduce it. As to Mary Jane, she is incorrigible, and my wife has given her notice, but there, again, I fail to see how you work it out.'

He chuckled to himself and rubbed his long, nervous hands together.

'It is simplicity itself,' said he; 'my eyes tell me that on the inside of your left shoe, just where the firelight strikes it, the leather is scored by six almost parallel cuts. Obviously they have been caused by someone who has very carelessly scraped round the edges of the sole in order to remove crusted mud from it. Hence, you see, my double deduction that you had been out in vile weather, and that you had a particularly malignant bootslitting specimen of the London slavey. As to your practice, if a gentleman walks into my rooms smelling of iodoform, with a black mark of nitrate of silver upon his right forefinger, and a bulge on the right side of his top-hat to show where he has secreted his stethoscope, I must be dull, indeed, if I do not pronounce him to be an active member of the medical profession.'

I could not help laughing at the ease with which he explained his process of deduction. **'When I hear you give your reasons,'** I remarked, **'the thing always appears to me to be so ridiculously simple** that I could easily do it myself, though at each successive instance of your reasoning I am baffled until you explain your process. And yet I believe that my eyes are as good as yours.' [*emphasis added*]

'Then how do you know?', Watson asks Holmes. 'I see it, I deduce it', says Holmes in reply. What made Holmes's explanations the superior ones, in Watson's eyes, was the fact that Holmes could, in an apparently scientific and law-like way, deduce so much about events from so few clues.

Sherlock Holmes and Father Brown differ in their detection styles but both have to 'give reasons' for their explanations. 'Then how did you know?' is a common refrain in detective fiction. Readers of detective fiction would not be happy if their favourite detective gave conclusions without reasons – without justifications for what constituted evidence and how evidence and conclusions fitted together.

But are there other styles of detection – Flashes of insight? Sudden guesses? Intuition? With no link to evidence at all?

Dirk Gently from Douglas Adams's *Dirk Gently's Holistic Detective Agency* is a good example of a detective who is not interested in the accounts people give him or in logical causal explanations of events. Dirk Gently's primary concern is with the 'fundamental interconnectedness of all things' – thus the 'holistic' in the title of Gently's detective agency: 'We solve the *whole* crime. We find the *whole* person' (Adams, 1987: 111). Dirk Gently tries to solve crimes with no reference to the logical connection between events, as in this scene with his secretary Miss Pearce.

He thrust a piece of paper across the desk.
She picked it up and looked at it. Then she turned it round and looked at it again.

She looked at the other side and then she put it down.

'Well?' demanded Dirk. 'What do you make of it? Tell me!'

Miss Pearce sighed.

'It's a lot of meaningless squiggles done in blue felt tip on a piece of typing paper,' she said. 'It looks like you did them yourself.'

'No!' barked Dirk, 'Well, yes,' he admitted, 'but only because I believe that is the answer to the problem!'

'What problem?'

'The problem,' insisted Dirk, slapping the table, 'of the conjuring trick! I told you!'

'Yes, Mr Gently, several times. I think it was just a conjuring trick. You see them on the telly.'

'With this difference – that this one was completely impossible!'

'Couldn't have been impossible or he wouldn't have done it. Stands to reason.'

'Exactly!' said Dirk excitedly. 'Exactly! Miss Pearce, you are a lady of rare perception and insight.'

'Thank you, sir, can I go now?'

'Wait! I haven't finished yet! Not by a long way, not by a bucketful! You have demonstrated to me the depth of your perception and insight, allow me to demonstrate mine!'

Miss Pearce slumped patiently in her seat.

'I think,' said Dirk, 'you will be impressed. Consider this. An intractable problem. In trying to find the solution to it I was going round and round in little circles in my mind, over and over the same maddening things. Clearly I wasn't going to be able to think of anything else until I had the answer, but equally clearly I would have to think of something else if I was ever going to get the answer. How to break this circle? Ask me how.'

'How?' said Miss Pearce obediently, but without enthusiasm.

'By writing down what the answer is!' exclaimed Dirk. 'And here it is!' he slapped the piece of paper triumphantly and sat back with a satisfied smile.

Miss Pearce looked at it dumbly.

'With the result,' continued Dirk, 'that I am now able to turn my mind to fresh and intriguing problems, like, for instance . . .'

He took the piece of paper, covered with its aimless squiggles and doodlings, and held it up to her.

'What language,' he said in a low, dark voice, 'is this written in?'

Miss Pearce continued to look at it dumbly.

Dirk flung the piece of paper down, put his feet up on the table, and threw his head back with his hands behind it.

'You see what I have done?' he asked the ceiling, which seemed to flinch slightly at being yanked so suddenly into the conversation. 'I have transformed the problem from an intractably difficult and possibly quite insoluble conundrum into a mere linguistic puzzle. 'Albeit', he muttered, after a long moment of silent pondering, 'an intractably difficult and possibly insoluble one.'

He swung back to gaze intently at Janice Pearce.

'Go on,' he urged, 'say that it's insane – but it might just work!'

Janice Pearce cleared her throat.

'It's insane,' she said, 'trust me.'

(Used by permission)

Dirk Gently sees a mystery where others do not. He provides meaningless answers to that mystery. His secretary does not accept that there is a mystery or the need for a solution. 'It's insane', says Miss Pearce. This is of course a part of the humour of this novel. Gently is an exaggerated example of the role that 'gut feelings', 'guessing' and 'lateral thinking' play in detective fiction. Guessing plays an important part in social science research, as we will see later.

Dirk Gently, like Sherlock Holmes, believes that it is possible to explain events by reference to 'wholes' – to interconnected laws that govern – on the surface – seemingly unrelated events. Gently, like Holmes, held that if you knew one link in the causal chain then you could find the 'whole'. This model of detection is similar to the 'nomothetic' model in social science research. A **nomothetic model** is a macro, probabilistic, approach to analysing what happens in society. The aim in the nomothetic model is to identify general classes of actions or events in society and not to show all the individual unique events that may lie behind them. The nomothetic model of research is often contrasted with **idiographic** models in social science, which analyse all the micro events behind a social phenomenon (Babbie, 1986: 53–55). Father Brown's inquiries are idiographic in nature. He looks at all the micro events associated with a murder mystery.

Both models of inquiry – nomothetic and idiographic – seek to explain what is happening. Both models must be grounded in 'everyday life'. The art of the detective and the social scientist, of course, is in the ability to identify important events and to explain the relationships between them. Father Brown's question 'But what happened then?' is the sign that an inquiry – an investigation – has started. A good detective and a good social scientist needs to know what, who, how and when to investigate. A good social scientist needs a research design.

KNOWING WHAT TO RESEARCH

Exploration, Description and Explanation

In the murder mystery *Cause of Death* Dr Kay Scarpetta, a medical examiner 'detective', is called out to a strange drowning in a naval shipyard for decommissioned naval ships and submarines. The first reaction of those investigating the incident was that it was simply a drowning: 'He probably just drowned,' Green was saying. 'Almost every diving death I've seen was a drowning. You die in water as shallow as this, that's what it's going to be' (Cornwell, 1997: 14).

Scarpetta, however, avoids 'closure' – premature finishing of the case. She takes the unusual step of diving to the body to investigate what has happened – to satisfy her own curiosity about what happened. She finds the air hose tangled on the side of an old ship but decides that the diver could have rectified this problem relatively easily. Scarpetta, after conducting the postmortem, finds that there is also cyanide in the body. The murder mystery gets more and more complex as the novel progresses, leading ultimately to a major conspiracy to take over a nuclear power plant.

Scarpetta explores, describes and then explains what is happening. Social science research sometimes involves all three kinds of research and sometimes only one. Exploratory research in social science is valuable when a researcher wants to study a new area and/or to test methods, such as surveys and survey questions, for investigating that area. Descriptive research is one of the most common forms of research in social science research. The census and surveys of public opinion are examples of descriptive research. The census, for example, provides an overview of demographics (e.g. gender, income) of a whole population. Public opinion polls show what people's voting intentions might be. A descriptive study may raise issues that need explaining. Explanatory research, however, reports not just 'what is happening' but 'why'. Let's look briefly at some descriptive and explanatory studies on the sociology of news and the journalism profession.

In January 1993 John Henningham published preliminary findings from a national survey of 1,068 Australian journalists, *The Hack's Progress* (1993: 45). The composite picture of a journalist, he said,

> is very different from the stereotype of middle-aged dissipation. The closer image is a 1990s yuppie. The survey shows that the typical journalist is male, young, and ambitious, with a middle-class, Anglo-Saxon background. There is an increasing chance that the journalist had a tertiary education and is likely to be well paid, content, committed to the career and optimistic about the future of the media. . . . About 37 per cent say they are more likely to vote Labor, with 29 per cent Liberal and 2 per cent National. The lean to the left is not a matter of background: most journalists come from middle-class families, with fewer than three out of 10 from blue-collar homes. Only one in 10 had parents in primary industry – cause for rural people to continue their complaints of limited and supposedly unsympathetic coverage of their problems. The churches might also argue under representation, with 74 per cent of journalists uninvolved in religion. Only 19 per cent of journalists were born overseas and almost all of them came from an Anglo-Celtic background. Fewer than 3 per cent of journalists are non-Caucasian.
>
> Women hold one in three jobs, but this is an advance on the early 1970s, when the ratio was one-in-10. Predictably, while 72 per cent of women say it is harder for females to advance their careers, only 39 per cent of male journalists agree. Women have an average of 27, against 37 for men. The combined median is 32, young enough to explain some of the optimism found in the survey.

The most extensive national survey of journalists ever undertaken is that done by Johnstone, Slawski and Bowman in the United States in 1971 and published in 1976. They surveyed 1,313 journalists by telephone from a national sample of 1,550. The authors estimate that fewer than half (45.7 per cent) of the 153,000 persons who reported themselves as 'editors or reporters' in the 1970 census were employed full-time in the American news media.

They estimated the total full-time editorial manpower in English-language news media in the United States at 69,500 and said that three-quarters of them were employed in print media, about 20 per cent in broadcast media and about 5 per cent in wire services at the time of their survey. More than half were employed by daily newspapers. Although they estimated that freelancers might contribute up to 100,000 stories a week to the news media, they did not include freelancers.

Johnstone, Slawski and Bowman found their 70,000 US journalists to be overwhelmingly young, urban, mobile and male – just as in Australia. They also found that their journalists did not conform to the stereotype of hard-drinking, callous and isolated creeps. In fact, they came from the same social strata as those in charge of the economic and political systems. There were few recruits from the working class.

Journalists did not *have* to have a degree to be a journalist but in fact 86 per cent of US journalists had attended college for one or more years, about 60 per cent were graduates and more than 18 per cent had done postgraduate work. Although most studied journalism more than any other specific subject, journalism majors were outnumbered by about 2 to 1 by persons with other kinds of college training. The other subjects most in demand were political science and government.

Johnstone, Slawski and Bowman's national survey of 1971 was replicated in 1982–3 by David Weaver and Cleveland Wilhoit (1986). In the years between 1971 and 1983 the USA had been involved in the Vietnam War, *All The President's Men* had exposed the criminal behaviour of Nixon and his aides in the White House, films such as *Absence of Malice* had questioned the ethics of journalists, the American media had been faced with a series of astronomical libel judgements, Janet Cooke had been awarded a Pulitzer Prize for a *Washington Post* story which she had faked and public confidence in the press had been eroded. Nevertheless, there was a 125 per cent increase in journalism and mass communication enrolments between 1971 and 1985.

By 1983 there were an estimated 112,072 journalists in the United States. Weaver and Wilhoit surveyed 1,001 of them. They found the typical journalist to be a politically moderate, 32-year-old, college-educated, white Protestant who earned $19,000 a year. The proportion of women had increased from 20 per cent in 1971 to 34 per cent in 1983. Two out of three journalists saw themselves as middle-of-the-road politically, 22 per cent saw themselves as left of centre and 18 per cent to the right. This was interesting because shortly before the Weaver and Wilhoit study was published, Lichter, Rothman and Lichter published their survey of 'elite' journalists – those working on 10 major news outlets – and said one out of two were left-of-centre, if the centre is defined as American businessmen. Their journalists were more likely than the national sample to see their role as challenging government. The Weaver and Wilhoit national sample were more moderate: most saw their role as being 'interpretive'. The next biggest proportion saw their role as disseminating information. Only a small proportion espoused the adversary role. In 1971, 58 per cent were college graduates whereas in 1983, 70 per cent were and more than half of those majored in journalism or communications. Generally, journalists earned less in real dollars than they did in 1971. Most said they heard more about their work from readers and viewers than from colleagues. When they studied another sample of 1,400 journalists in the 1990s they found that journalists had less autonomy than reported in the earlier studies and less job satisfaction. The proportion of journalists planning to leave the profession was double that of the 1983 studies. But the typical American journalist remained a married white male in his thirties, with a bachelor's degree (Weaver and Wilhoit, 1996).

Similar findings emerge from the British studies. In his *Journalism Recruitment and Training: Problems in Professionalization* Oliver Boyd-Barrett reports a 1969 survey of 99 trainee journalists in the two largest training centres (1970: 181–201). More than half of them came from lower-middle and upper-middle white-collar backgrounds and nine came from senior executive–managerial–professional backgrounds. About half could qualify for entrance to a university and he cites estimates that graduates comprise from 6 to 15 per cent of the total intake of recruits to journalism each year. Most (62 per cent) of those in his sample who were employed by newspapers obtained their first job by writing letters on their own initiative to one or several newspapers and another 25 per cent answered press advertisements.

Boyd-Barrett's work also had an explanatory element. He investigated the reasons for choosing journalism as a career: it was seen as a non-routine, non-conventional, sociable occupation by 35 per cent of respondents; it was the most desirable occupation available to 29 per cent; it was seen as creative by 16 per cent and more than 75 per cent wanted to write a book (a novel in most cases); it was seen as self-educational by 5 per cent; as a 'bridging occupation' to a better job by 3 per cent; and as a public service occupation by 1 per cent. In spite of the aspirations for the non-routine, non-conventional and the creative, in practice the young journalists spent a quarter or more of their work time at desk work or office work and most of their outside work on covering routine, predictable events. Feature writing accounted for only 10 per cent of total time. Nevertheless, they felt little dissatisfaction with the organization of their work or its opportunities. Most of them wanted to go into feature writing, general reporting or special writing which they saw as offering more opportunities for self-expression and initiative.

Boyd-Barrett (1970: 60–4) says that most British recruits to journalism begin on weekly provincial newspapers and that juniors made up about two-fifths of the journalists on these papers in each of the years 1964–7. Almost all start as general reporters and their first chance to specialize is usually in sport. Although more than 60 per cent of national newspaper journalists in Britain were over 35, the belief was widely held that 'on your 35th birthday they push you down the rubbish chute'. It was also widely asserted that many journalists were sacked but Tunstall (1970) could find little evidence of this for the period 1965–8.

An understanding of the demographics of the journalism profession as well as journalists' motivations for joining the profession combines descriptive and explanatory aspects of social science research. The 'what' of the research and the 'why' of the research overlap. In the surveys cited above it is possible to gain an overview of who journalists are and to discover trends in the journalism profession, including journalists' attitudes towards journalism.

Topics of Research

Knowing what to research, knowing the purpose of the research, is key to the first steps in a research design. Knowing whether the research is exploratory, descriptive or explanatory is a part of knowing what to research. The topics of social science research range from description – describing who the people or social groups are – to explanation – explaining why those people or social groups think or behave the way they do.

Analysing how people or social groups think and behave includes analysis of attitudes, beliefs, personality traits and other factors associated with motivation. Analysing how people or social groups behave includes analysis of the actual actions. Table 2.1, for example, tells us what is happening with Western Samoan television behaviour, but it does not tell us why the Samoans changed their behaviour. Why did they stop weaving mats? Was television the cause?

What people do and what they say they do can also differ to a great degree. In 1934 Lapiere travelled with a Chinese couple to 66 hotels, auto-

TABLE 2.1   Impact of television on Western Samoan evening activities, 4–10 pm

	% of time spent	
	Without TV	With TV
Prayers	6	4
Eating	17	10
Talking/Discussion	30	9
Story telling/Singing	15	3
Visiting friends/ Community activities	22	4
Playing cards/ Weaving mats	10	0
Watching TV	0	70

Source: Martin (1987: 3–21)

mobile camps, tourist homes, and 184 restaurants and cafes in the United States. The Chinese couple were accepted with open arms. Lapiere then sent questionnaires to all the places he visited, asking them if they would accept Chinese as guests. Ninety per cent replied 'No' (Deutscher, 1973).

Detectives like the medical examiner Kay Scarpetta go through all the steps of modern social science research. There is an exploratory element – seeing whether there is a suspicious death; there is a descriptive element – describing what actually happened to the dead person; and there is an explanatory element – the reasons for the person's murder by cyanide. Scarpetta is interested in what people tell her but she is also interested in the actual behaviour of the people she talks to.

Knowing what to research involves decisions on exploration, description and explanation as well as decisions about the topic of the research itself. These decisions will form part of a research design. Knowing whom to research is also an important part of research design. Knowing whom is not simply a matter of which people might be relevant to a study, but which units of analysis.

KNOWING WHOM TO RESEARCH

Units of Analysis

Surveys on journalism as a profession involve individual journalists as the unit of analysis – each journalist is asked a question in a survey. The individual journalist is also a member of a larger grouping – the profession itself. If we make the explanatory statement 'educated men are more likely than educated women to be journalists', then we are working at the level of the individual as the unit of analysis. If we make the descriptive statement that 'the typical American journalist is a married white male in his thirties, with a bachelor's degree', then we are also dealing with the individual as the unit of analysis. However, if we said that journalists are more likely than accountants to be tertiary educated, then we would be using the group as the unit of analysis.

The social science researcher also has to decide who counts as a 'journalist'. This is especially important if we are drawing a 'sample' of journalists for investigation. We will deal with samples and populations later, but there are important issues associated with the definition of a 'journalist'. Is a journalist anyone who belongs to the journalists' association or is it anyone who writes a story for a publication (a local newsletter?). Is anyone who runs their own website a journalist?

The 'who' of research involves identifying the individuals who might be relevant to a study and the social groups to which they belong. Sherlock Holmes did this in his own way when he told Watson how he identified him. 'As to your practice, if a gentleman walks into my rooms smelling of iodoform, with a black mark of nitrate of silver upon his right forefinger, and a bulge on the right side of his top-hat to show where he has secreted his stethoscope, I must be dull, indeed, if I do not pronounce him to be an active member of the medical profession.'

In social science research it is essential that you identify what your unit of analysis is. Is it criminals or crimes? Is it journalists or journalism? Understanding your units of analysis forms part of your decisions on research design. Poor definition of the unit of analysis and poor selection of those units raise questions about the external validity of a study – can the results be generalized from a sample to all the units of analysis you are studying? Your literature review will also help you to clarify the what and the who of your study.

KNOWING HOW TO RESEARCH

Literature Review

Coming up with good topics in social science research is not easy. Narrowing the topic – giving it a decent focus and decent definition – is even more difficult. One of the most complex research topics this century has been 'Does media violence cause violent behaviour?' Popular concern about the relationship between media and behaviour has been ongoing. In 1993, international news agencies reported the murder of a four–year-old English boy, James Bulger, by two 10-year-olds who kidnapped him from a shopping centre and took him to a railway line. The four-year-old suffered 30 blows inflicting 22 injuries to his head, another 20 to his body. Bags containing 27 bloodstained bricks were also shown to the jury together with a 22 kg railway bolt used in the attack. The 10-year-old boys had watched over 300 adult violent videos in the previous six months.

News media and the popular imagination often put media violence and violent behaviour together in a causal relationship. But a causal relationship has been difficult to measure. Social science research has swung backwards and forwards from 'no effect' to 'powerful effects' and back again. Violent video games are one of the latest research topics.

'Computer games don't trigger aggression: report', said The West Australian, (December 4, 1999: 14). This five-year study, supported by the Australian government, concluded that 'Computer games do not promote aggressive behaviour and are less disturbing for children than movies, according to a new report. They are not addictive, nor do they ruin family life, impair school performance or cause health problems' (Durkin and Aisbett, 1999).

Cumberbatch and Howitt undertook a 'state of the science' review of media effects in 1989. They covered research into specific effects in areas such as women and sex roles, race and racism, age and ageism, disablement, alcohol, prosocial issues, sex and violence. Their conclusion was that the 'history of mass communication research is conspicuously lacking in any clear evidence on the precise influence of the mass media. Theories abound, examples multiply, but convincing facts that specific media content is reliably associated with particular effects have proved quite elusive' (Cumberbatch and Howitt, 1989: 25).

One of the reasons for the difficulty in establishing cause and effect, according to Cumberbatch and Howitt, is that isolating the contribution mass media make to problems such as violence is extremely difficult because social perceptions about these phenomena are deeply embedded and often difficult to define.

Lowrey and DeFleur (1983: 339) in their review of research argued that there are three general possibilities which describe a possible relationship between viewing media violence and aggressive behaviour:

1   The viewing of violence leads to aggressive tendencies.
2   Aggressive tendencies lead to the choosing of violence viewing.
3   Aggressive tendencies and the viewing of violence are both products of some third condition or set of conditions.

Lowrey and DeFleur's conclusion is that 'regular or frequent viewing of violent television programs may cause aggressive behaviour' (1983: 341).

An analysis of other people's work, as the media and violence research demonstrates, requires a critical eye. Stern and Kalof (1996), summarized in Figure 2.1, provide a simple guide to checking 'statements of fact' – whether statements constitute genuine evidence.

Some statements by authors are unsupported assertions. Simply saying that media violence leads to violent behaviour is an unsupported assertion. Simply referring to an author who says that media violence leads to violent behaviour is certainly trying to support the statement, but it is an 'appeal to

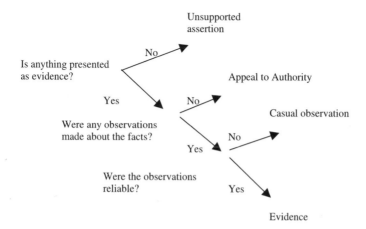

FIGURE 2.1   *From assertions to evidence (used by permission)*

authority' rather than substantial evidence. If the author referred to has substantiated his or her observations in a reliable manner, then we are getting closer to evidence.

A literature review – seeing what journal articles, books and other sources say about previous and contemporary research on the topic – is essential for planning a research design. Like a compass, a literature review gives the researcher a bearing on what has been done. It also assists conceptualization and measurement in research design.

For example, violence as we all know is real, but how does a researcher measure it? Sherman and Dominick (1986) attempted to measure the occurrence of violence in music videos. In their content analysis of violence in music videos it was found that women, older adults and nonwhites are more likely to be represented as aggressors than victims. 'Aggressors and victims were most likely to fall in the young adult age range (18–34). Interestingly, older adults (35–54) were nearly twice as likely to be aggressors as victims. For children, an opposite trend was noted: they were twice as likely to be the targets as the agents of aggression' (1986: 86–87). The unit of analysis in Sherman and Dominick's content analysis was the 'concept video'. For measurement of violence they used Gerbner's definition of a violent act as an 'overt expression of physical force with or without a weapon, against self or other, compelling action against one's will on pain of being hurt or killed or actually killing or hurting' (Gerbner, cited in Sherman and Dominick, 1986: 83–4). Independent coders then categorized aggressive and violent content by the type of violence (pushing, punching, slapping, gunshot, etc.), whether the aggressor was an individual or group, the sex, ethnic background and age of the victim, outcome of the aggression (death, injury, no effect) and whether the violence was portrayed realistically or unrealistically (1986: 84).

Your reaction to Sherman and Dominick's definition of 'violence' might be that it is too narrow – surely there is emotional violence? psychological violence? what about shouting? Once you start raising these types of questions you are querying the validity of the definitions being used – the construct validity and the internal validity of the study in question. These are exactly the types of questions you should raise about definitions in a study because it is these definitions that affect the measurement. Poor definitions mean poor measurement.

The goal of a study should always be clearly stated. Spillman and Everington (1989), for example, provided uncomplicated sentences to describe their study: 'The purpose of this study was to investigate whether the thin image presented by media today is consistent with earlier body-image stereotypes or whether current stereotypes are different. That is, is this image now perceived by college students as possessing more desirable characteristics?'

Spillman and Everington (1989) found in their literature review that researchers have consistently reported stereotypical behavioural and personality traits associated with each of the three different body-build somatypes of endomorph, mesomorph and ectomorph. The most favourable traits have been assigned to the mesomorphic body build and the least favorable to the ectomorphic and endomorphic builds. Their sample was responses from 234 undergraduate students to a questionnaire. Each student was asked to fill out a questionnaire of 10 questions describing themselves (age, sex, weight range, height range, class, and school designation). The next 24 questions required an individual to assign a behavioural characteristic to one of three female silhouettes. Spillman and Everington (1989) found in their results that the very thin body image, the ectomorph, was the most preferred somatype.

Secondary Analysis

Previous studies like Spillman and Everington's can be replicated – done again – in different contexts or at different points in time – to see what is happening. Indeed, previous data can be re-analysed by other researchers. This is called secondary analysis. The wealth of survey data in modern societies, whether census, opinion poll, or other survey data, makes secondary analysis a common and economical method of research.

Secondary analysis may also form part of exploratory work in a study – for example identifying the characteristics of the people you are studying from previous survey data. If the same methodology for collecting data has been used over long periods of time, then useful comparison can be made. Time is, indeed, an important factor in social science research design. A thorough grounding in the literature – the journal articles, books, reports – associated with a research topic provides direction on how the research might be conducted. Knowing when to research is also a critical dimension of research design.

KNOWING WHEN TO RESEARCH

The Importance of Time

Sherlock Holmes, quite rightly, calls his work 'cases'. They are case studies that investigate 'what is happening'. It is an investigation of one crime at a particular point of time. Holmes's only long-term criminal investigation involves his nemesis, Professor Moriarty – the criminal genius.

Exploring, describing and explaining in quantitative social science research requires a research design. Decisions on conceptualization, measurement and who is to be researched also require a research design. Time is important in a research design when the researcher wants to make comparisons. A simple case study involves looking at a single phenomenon at a particular point in time. A longitudinal study involves investigating a phenomenon or different groups over time, to see if there are any relevant changes. For example, there have been changes in the demographics of the journalism profession over time. Time is also relevant to experiments. An experiment is a very controlled attempt to see whether specific independent variables (assumed causes) are related to specific dependent variables (assumed effects). The researcher tries to manipulate the environment in an experiment to see what is happening. We will return to the idea of 'independent variables' in Chapter 3. Table 2.2 gives an overview of the general options in research design.

Exploratory and descriptive research often use cross-sectional designs. A British or US census, for example, is cross-sectional and describes the population at a given point of time. Explanatory research can use cross-sectional designs. A study designed to examine the influence of religious affiliation on voting, for example, could be done at a particular point in time. The problem with such 'snapshot' research, if not replicated, is that it cannot take into account changes over time. Longitudinal research solves this problem by enabling comparison of the same groups and the same phenomena over time. TV ratings, for example, involve the establishment

TABLE 2.2   Time and research design

Simple Case Study/Cross-Sectional Design

What's happening?

(A)

Longitudinal Study/Trends Studies/Panel Studies

Has there been a change in A over time?

(A)   (A)

Time 1   Time 2

Comparison

Are A and B different?

(A)

(B)

Longitudinal Comparison

Are A and B different over time?

(A)   (A)

Time 1   Time 2

(B)   (B)

Time 1   Time 2

Longitudinal Comparison

Are A and B different over time because of the independent variable?

Experimental Group
X (independent variable) ⟶   (A)   (A)

Time 1   Time 2

Control Group   (B)   (B)

Time 1   Time 2

Adapted from Bouma (1993: 111). (Used by permission).

of 'panels', thousands of households, that are monitored regularly by ratings agencies.

RESEARCH DESIGN

We now have a rough checklist of the key elements of a research design. Great ideas are important in social science research, just as they are in detective fiction, but good ideas must be backed up by good design. Good design assists not only the investigation but the administration of quantitative research. It is very easy to underestimate the practical, administrative, side of organizing, collecting and analysing evidence. Table 2.3 outlines the key elements associated with research planning.

Many of the concepts in Table 2.3 have not yet been introduced, but they do provide you with a roadmap to what is required. We will return to all the major concepts as the book proceeds.

SUMMARY

Detectives try to make sense of what has happened, what is happening or what is going to happen, in the world about them. They use different methodologies and methods to make sense of, or add intelligibility to, the evidence that faces them. They are also required to show how they came to their conclusions and why one conclusion should be accepted rather than another. Social science research, similarly, is public. It is required to demonstrate its findings and to make itself open to critique and review.

There is the possibility of error in social science research. These errors can be errors of human prejudice, errors of ego involvement (Holmes said he tried to put prejudice aside); errors in observation (Watson was chastised for not observing at all!); and premature closure of inquiry (Holmes was scathing about police prejudging crimes, Scarpetta never closed off investigations too quickly). There is also the possibility of overgeneralization (Father Brown never made wild conclusions from the evidence).

The extracts from the works of Chesterton, Conan Doyle and Adams show that different processes of reasoning and explanation occur in detective fiction. These processes of reasoning have their parallel in quantitative research. Social scientists, like fictional detectives, have *theories* and *hypotheses* which they test against the evidence. They also have *methods* by which they collect and analyse that evidence. Theories, hypotheses and methods are integral to research and make research systematic.

Of course, there are different theories and different methods in social science just as there are different styles of detection in fictional detective novels. But common to all detective fiction, and social science, is the requirement to explain what counts as evidence, and how conclusions fit

TABLE 2.3   *Organizing a quantitative research study*

PROBLEM
What is the goal of the research?
What is the problem, issue, or critical focus to be researched?
What are the important terms? What do they mean?
What is the significance of the problem?
Do you want to test a theory?
Do you want to extend a theory?
Do you want to test competing theories?
Do you want to test a method?
Do you want to replicate a previous study?
Do you want to correct previous research that was conducted in an inadequate manner?
Do you want to resolve inconsistent results from earlier studies?
Do you want to solve a practical problem?
Do you want to add to the body of knowledge in another manner?

REVIEW OF LITERATURE
What does previous research reveal about the problem?
What is the theoretical framework for the investigation?
Are there complementary or competing theoretical frameworks?
What are the hypotheses and research questions that have emerged from the literature review?

SAMPLE
Who (what) will provide (constitute) the data for the research?
What is the population being studied?
Who will be the participants for the research?
What sampling technique will be used?
What materials and information are necessary to conduct the research?
How will they be obtained?
What special problems can be anticipated in acquiring needed materials and information?
What are the limitations in the availability and reporting of materials and information?

METHOD
What methods or techniques will be used to collect the data? (This holds for applied and non-applied research)
What procedures will be used to apply the methods or techniques?
What are the limitations of these methods?
What factors will affect the study's internal and external validity?
Will any ethical principles be jeopardized?

DATA ANALYSIS
How will data be analysed?
What statistics will be used?
What criteria will be used to determine whether hypotheses are supported?
What was discovered (about the goal, data, method, and data analysis) as a result of doing preliminary work (if conducted)?

CONCLUDING INFORMATION
How will the final research report be organized? (Outline)
What sources have you examined thus far that pertain to your study? (Reference list)
What additional information does the reader need?
What time frame (deadlines) have you established for collecting, analysing and presenting data? (Timetable)

Adapted from Rubin et al. (1990)

the evidence. Logical argument based on sound empirical evidence for detectives and social scientists alike is superior to argument based on false evidence, or no evidence at all. Social scientists are detectives. They collect *empirical* evidence from the social world around them and make decisions about that evidence. 'Empirical research' in this case simply means research *based on evidence from the real world* in contrast to *theoretical*, which refers to ideas that are abstract or purely analytical. 'A theory remains theoretical until it is tested against the real world, with empirical evidence' (McNeill, 1985: 2).

We will use the detective theme throughout this book on quantitative methods. Quantitative methods and statistics in social science are about logical inquiry. The different types of logic and the different types of personality in detective fiction and social science are often the same. You will find quirky characters in both types of detection, including the Dirk Gently.

We will examine in depth the logic behind the styles of reasoning of detectives like Father Brown and Sherlock Holmes and the nature of the continuum between qualitative and quantitative. We will give examples of famous detective stories of social science – showing how inquiries were started, investigated, and concluded. We will, finally, provide you with some important tools of analysis – basic statistics.

The Statistical Inquirer

The Statistical Inquirer multimedia courseware provided on the CD-ROM introduces you to descriptive statistics. The step-by-step lessons cover the library, the concept of variables, measures of centrality, variance, correlation and regression, as well as the idea of statistical inference. These lessons are designed to reinforce what is covered in this text. Short videos, using LotusScreencam, provide a brief introduction to SPSS. A dataset from Patrick Rawstorne's doctoral study on subjective computer anxiety, Predicting and Explaining the use of Information Technology with Value Expectancy Models of Behaviour in Contexts of Mandatory Use, has been provided for practice. An Unsolved Mystery also gives you the opportunity to test your basic statistics skills.

MAIN POINTS

- There is a logic to social science inquiry. Quantitative social scientific inquiry requires evidence that is observable and testable. Researchers must give explanations for their conclusions. Social science research is public. This assists in avoiding bias in research.
- A research design is the guide to how the research was constructed and carried out.

- Explanations in social science can be 'nomothetic', dealing with the larger contexts in which social phenomena occur, or 'idiographic', dealing with unique events. 'Data', however, is not 'pregiven' in the social sciences – it is a part of processes of interpretation in society. Definitions of 'violence' are already affected, for example, by perceptions in society of what violence is.
- Social science research can be exploratory, descriptive or explanatory. Exploratory research is used for testing new ideas or areas of research and/or testing methods used to collect data. Descriptive research, like TV ratings, describes 'what is' and provides an overview of a phenomenon. Explanatory research seeks to explain 'why'. 'Why' questions tend to be theory questions.
- Units of analysis are part of 'what is counted' in quantitative research. This can be individuals or groups. It can also be items in a content analysis of a newspaper or a video.
- A literature review is a preliminary investigation of what has been done or what is being done in an area of study. It is essential to planning a study. As you can see from the brief overviews of journalism as a profession and the relationship between media and effects, there is a substantial amount of existing research in these areas of study.
- Secondary analysis is an economical way of finding out new things from existing data.
- Time is a major factor in developing a research design. Research can be conducted once, at a particular point in time, or over time. Trend studies and panels are longitudinal and allow comparison over time. Experiments are the most controlled of all research studies, allowing investigation of the impact of specific phenomena over a period of time.

REVIEW EXERCISES

1 Find two journal articles from a sociology, psychology or media journal that you think are examples of descriptive and explanatory research. Write a brief one-page summary of the research design.
2 Find a report on a research study in a newspaper, magazine or the internet that you think uses unsupported assertions, appeals to authority or casual observation (that do not appear to have been tested).
3 Classify the following statements as either unsupported assertion, appeal to authority, casual observation or evidence.

'I never met a person I did not like'
'Everyone knows that smoking causes lung cancer'
'According to Rogers (1970) opinion leaders have extraordinary influence over diffusion of innovations'

REFERENCES

Adams, D. (1987) *Dirk Gently's Holistic Detective Agency*. London: Heinemann.

Babbie, E. (1986) *The Practice of Social Research*. Belmont: Wadsworth.

Bouma, G.D. (1993) *The Research Process*. New York: Oxford.

Boyd-Barrett, O. (1970) 'Journalism recruitment and training: problems in professionalisation', in Jeremy Tunstall (ed.), *Media Sociology*. London: Constable.

Chesterton, G.K. (1987) *The Complete Father Brown: the enthralling adventures of fiction's best-loved amateur sleuth*. London: Penguin.

Cornwell, P. (1997) *Cause of Death*. London: Warner.

Cumberbatch, G. and Howitt, D. (1989) *A Measure of Uncertainty: The effects of the mass media*. London: J. Libbey.

Deutscher, I. (1973) *What We Say, What We Do: sentiments and acts*. Glenview, IL: Scott, Foresman.

Doyle, Arthur Conan (1952) *The Complete Sherlock Holmes*. Garden City, New York: Doubleday.

Durkin, K. and Aisbett, K. (1999) *Computer Games and Australians Today*. Office of Film and Literature Classification.

Henningham, J. (1981) 'The television journalist: A profile', *Media Information Australia*, 22: 5.

Henningham, J. (ed.) (1990) *Issues in Australian Journalism*. Melbourne: Longman Cheshire.

Henningham, J. (1993) 'The hack's progress', *Time*, 11 January: 45.

Henningham, J. (1996) 'Australian journalists' views on professional associations', *Asia Pacific Media Educator* (1): 144–52.

Hudson, W.J. (1964) 'The education of a journalist in Australia', in E.L. French (ed.) *Melbourne Studies in Education 1963*. Melbourne: Melbourne University Press. pp. 321-47.

Hudson, W.J. (1964) 'Status of the metropolitan daily journalist in Australia', *The Australian Journal of Social Issues*, 2 (2).

Johnstone, J.W.C, Slawski, E.J. and Bowman, W.W. (1976) *The News People: A Sociological Portrait of American Journalists and Their Work*. Urbana, IL: University of Illinois Press.

Jones, R.L. and Swanson, C.E. (1954) 'Small-city daily newspapermen: their abilities and interests', *Journalism Quarterly*, 31: 38–55.

Judd, R.P. (1961) 'The newspaper reporter in a suburban city', *Journalism Quarterly*, 38: 35-43.

Lichter, S.R., Rothman, S. and Lichter, L.S. (1986) *Media Elite: America's new power-brokers*. Bethesda, MD: Ahler and Ahler.

Lowrey, S. and DeFleur, M.L. (1983) *Milestones in Mass Communication Research*. New York: Longman.

Martin, A. (1987) 'Media and social change – with special reference to television', *Pacific Islands Communication Journal*, 15 (1): 3–21.

McNeill, P. (1985) *Research Methods*. London: Tavistock.

Rubin, R.B., Rubin, A.M. and Piele, J. (1990) *Communication Research: Strategies and Sources* (2nd edn). Belmont, CA: Wadsworth.

Sherman, B.L. and Dominick, J.R. (1986) 'Violence and sex in music videos: TV and rock 'n' roll', *Journal of Communication*, 36 (1): 79–93.

Spillman, D. and Everington, C. (1989) 'Somatypes revisited: have the media changed our perception of the female body image?', *Psychological Reports*, 64: 887–90.

Stern, P.C. and Kalof, L. (1996) *Evaluating Social Science Research*. New York: Oxford.

Tunstall, J. (1970) *Media Sociology*. London: Constable.

Weaver, D.H. and Wilhoit, G.C. (1986) *The American Journalist: A portrait of U.S. News People and Their Work*, Malwah, NJ: Lawrence Erlbaum.

Weaver, D.H. and Wilhoit, G.C. (1996) *The American Journalist in the 1990s: U.S. News People at the End of an Era*. Malwah, NJ: Lawrence Erlbaum.

White, D.M. (1950) 'The gatekeeper: a case study in the selection of news', *Journalism Quarterly*, 27: 383–90.

3
Defining the Inquiry

'Then how do you know?'

'I never guess'

Sherlock Holmes, *The Sign of Four*

Sherlock Holmes realized that what often led the police of his day astray was their tendency to adopt theories of a crime based on the wrong facts. There is nothing more deceptive than an obvious fact, says Holmes.

> 'By an examination of the ground I gained the trifling details which I gave to that imbecile Lestrade, as to the personality of the criminal.'
> 'But how did you gain them?'
> 'You know my method. It is founded upon the observation of trifles.' (*The Boscombe Valley Mystery*)

Sherlock Holmes said that he did not guess. He relied on observations and he had a method for analysing those observations. 'Seeing' was not enough for Holmes. Accurate observations were essential for his method.

> 'You see, but you do not observe [said Holmes to Watson]. The distinction is clear. For example, you have frequently seen the steps which lead up from the hall to this room.'
> 'Frequently.'
> 'How often?'
> 'Well, some hundreds of times.'
> 'Then how many are there?'
> 'How many? I don't know.'
> 'Quite so! You have not observed. And yet you have seen. That is just my point. Now, I know that there are seventeen steps, because I have both seen and observed.' (*A Scandal in Bohemia*)

Observations are the key to quantitative research methods. Measuring observations is the task of quantitative research. But knowing that your observations are quantifiable and constitute real evidence is no simple matter. In Chapter 2 we discovered that there is a range of ways of starting an inquiry and designing a quantitative research study. We also found that social scientists, like detectives, have different styles of reasoning about evidence and what constitutes evidence. Finding a clue is one thing. But making inferences, judgements, about the relevance of the clue is another matter. Holmes's criticism of the police is based on his judgement that the police not only missed the important clues but that their system for making judgements about clues was also wrong. Holmes criticized police methodology – their science for finding out, as well as their method – their actual techniques for recognizing and collecting clues. In this chapter we will explore the different styles of reasoning about evidence – methodology – and the systems of measurement that have been developed to quantify observations.

TOOLS OF METHODOLOGY

Holmes did not like theorizing – trying to provide explanations – without data. He took detection to be about observed data, deduction and prediction. His methods of detection, he said, were 'an impersonal thing – a thing beyond myself'. The great consulting detective's methods of detection entailed 'severe reasoning from cause to effect' and, according to him, were really the only notable feature about his cases. 'Crime is common. Logic is rare', said Holmes to Watson, berating his loyal partner for being too sensationalist in his accounts of the different cases. 'It is upon the logic rather than upon the crime that you should dwell.'

Holmes said that 'all life is a great chain, the nature of which is known whenever we are shown a single link' (*Study in Scarlet*). If you think that this statement sounds 'nomothetic', then you are correct. Holmes's confidence in his ability to show the 'great chain' even extended to attempts to read the train of thought of a person from their features, as was demonstrated to Dr Watson in the story of the *The Resident Patient*.

It had been a close, rainy day in October. Our blinds were half-drawn, and Holmes lay curled upon the sofa, reading and re-reading a letter which he had received by the morning post. For myself, my term of service in India had trained me to stand heat better than cold, and a thermometer of ninety was no hardship. But the paper was uninteresting. Parliament had risen. Everybody was out of town, and I yearned for the glades of the New Forest or the shingle of Southsea. A depleted bank account had caused me to postpone my holiday, and as to my companion, neither the country nor the sea presented the slightest attraction to him. He loved to lie in the very centre of five millions of people, with his filaments stretching out and running through them, responsive to every little rumour or suspicion of unsolved crime. Appreciation of nature found no place among his many gifts, and his only change was when he turned his mind from the evildoer of the town to track down his brother of the country.

Finding that Holmes was too absorbed for conversation, I had tossed aside the barren paper, and, leaning back in my chair I fell into a brown study. Suddenly my companion's voice broke in upon my thoughts.

'You are right, Watson,' said he. 'It does seem a very preposterous way of settling a dispute.'

'Most preposterous!' I exclaimed, and then, suddenly realizing how he had echoed the inmost thought of my soul, I sat up in my chair and stared at him in blank amazement.

'What is this, Holmes?' I cried. 'This is beyond anything which I could have imagined.'

He laughed heartily at my perplexity.

'You remember,' said he, 'that some little time ago, when I read you the passage in one of Poe's sketches, in which a close reasoner follows the unspoken thoughts of his companion, you were inclined to treat the matter as a mere tour de force of the author. On my remarking that I was constantly in the habit of doing the same thing you expressed incredulity.'

'Oh, no!'

'Perhaps not with your tongue, my dear Watson, but certainly with your eyebrows. So when I saw you throw down your paper and enter upon a train of thought, I was very happy to have the opportunity of reading it off, and eventually of breaking into it, as a proof that I had been in rapport with you.'

But I was still far from satisfied. 'In the example which you read to me,' said I, 'the reasoner drew his conclusions from the actions of the man whom he observed. If I remember right, he stumbled over a heap of stones, looked up at the stars, and so on. But I have been seated quietly in my chair, and what clues can I have given you?'

'You do yourself an injustice. The features are given to man as the means by which he shall express his emotions, and yours are faithful servants.'

'Do you mean to say that you read my train of thoughts from my features?'

'Your features, and especially your eyes. Perhaps you cannot yourself recall how your reverie commenced?'

'No, I cannot.'

'Then I will tell you. After throwing down your paper, which was the action which drew my attention to you, you sat for half a minute with a vacant expression. Then your eyes fixed themselves upon your newly framed picture of General Gordon, and I saw by the alteration in your face that a train of thought had been started. But it did not lead very far. Your eyes turned across to the unframed portrait of Henry Ward Beecher, which stands upon the top of your books. You then glanced up at the wall, and of course your meaning was obvious. You were thinking that if the portrait were framed it would just cover that bare space and correspond with Gordon's picture over there.'

'You have followed me wonderfully!' I exclaimed.

'So far I could hardly have gone astray. But now your thoughts went back to Beecher, and you looked hard across as if you were studying the character in his features. Then your eyes ceased to pucker, but you continued to look across, and your face was thoughtful. You were recalling the incidents of Beecher's career. I was well aware that you could not do this without thinking of the mission which he undertook on behalf of the North at the time of the Civil War, for I remember you expressing your passionate indignation at the way in which he was received by the more turbulent of our people. You felt so strongly about it that I knew you could not think of Beecher without thinking of that also. When a moment later I saw your eyes wander away from the picture, I suspected that your mind had now turned to the Civil War, and when I observed that your lips set, your eyes sparkled, and your hands clinched, I was positive that you were indeed thinking of the gallantry which was shown by both sides in that desperate struggle. But then, again, your face grew sadder; you shook your head. You were dwelling upon the sadness and horror and useless waste of life. Your hand stole towards your own old wound, and a smile quivered on your lips, which showed me that the ridiculous side of this method of settling international questions had forced itself upon your mind. At this point I agreed with you that it was preposterous, and was glad to find that all my deductions had been correct.

'Absolutely!' said I. 'And now that you have explained it, I confess that I am as amazed as before.'

'It was very superficial, my dear Watson, I assure you. I should not have intruded it upon your attention had you not shown some incredulity the other day. But the evening has brought a breeze with it. What do you say to a ramble through London?'

Sherlock Holmes did not have to *talk* to Watson to discover his thoughts and intentions. He could, he said, infer the thoughts, and their sequence, from specific non-verbal events. What strikes us with Holmes is his emphasis on cause and effect, and the treatment of his observations and deductions as though they were scientific. Indeed, Holmes is the epitome of the scientific detective. He wrote an article for a magazine about science and deduction called 'The Book of Life' and a monograph outlining his scientific method called *Upon the Distinction Between the Ashes of the Various Tobaccos: An Enumeration of 140 Forms of Cigar, Cigarette and Pipe Tobacco, with Coloured Plates Illustrating the Differences in the Ash*. It is precisely the scientific side of the cocaine-snorting Holmes that made him a hero of 19th and 20th century readers.

Styles of Reasoning (deduction, induction and abduction)

Holmes's reading of Watson's thoughts, however, is not, in fact, deduction. It is, in fact, a case of *abduction*, or guessing, as Umberto Eco (1983: 216), who wrote his own detective novel *The Name of the Rose*, has pointed out. 'Watson threw down his paper and then fixed the picture of General Gordon. This was undoubtedly *a fact*. That afterward he looked to another (unframed) portrait was another *fact*. That he could have thought of the relation between these two portraits can be a case of undercoded abduction, based on Holmes's knowledge of Watson's interest in interior decoration. But that, from this point on, Watson thought of the incidents of Beecher's career was undoubtedly a creative abduction . . . Holmes invented a story. It simply happened that that possible story was analogous to the actual one.'

Holmes, in short, *guessed*, but what is appealing to the reader is the fact that he guessed so well. For Eco, Holmes was 'meta-betting' – betting that the 'possible world' he has outlined – his guess – is the same as the 'real one' – Watson's actual thoughts. There is an important difference between Eco and Holmes on this point. Holmes thinks that his inferences – his deductions – about his observations can be referred back to a 'great chain' of causes and effects. Eco is saying that Holmes's guesses are not deductions.

Umberto Eco introduces the idea of *undercoded abduction,* which is, for all intents and purposes, the old idea of *induction.* He also uses the idea of *overcoded abduction,* which is the old idea of *deduction.* Creative abductions (or meta-abductions) for Eco are the big guesses. Detectives bet by meta-abduction, scientists test their abductions.

What Watson's account shows us is that Holmes used different kinds of logic – and guessing was one of them. For Holmes, all knowledge is derived from hypotheses, but a hypothesis is not always fully tested. Holmes indirectly acknowledges the more dangerous nature of hypothesis when he advocates the use of 'imagination' (*The Retired Colourman, Silver Blaze*), 'intuition' (*The Sign of Four*) and 'speculation' (*Hound of the Baskervilles*). Holmes is referring here to what C.S. Peirce called 'abduction' or 'retroduction'.

> Abduction makes its start from the facts, without, at the outset having any particular theory in view, though it is motivated by the feeling that a theory is needed to explain the surprising facts. Induction makes its start from a hypothesis which seems to recommend itself, without at the outset having any particular facts in view, though it feels the need of facts to support the theory. Abduction seeks a theory. Induction seeks for facts. In abduction the consideration of the facts suggests the hypothesis. In induction the study of the hypothesis suggests the experiments which bring to light the very facts to which the hypothesis had pointed (cited in Sebeok and Umiker-Sebeok, 1983: 25).

Peirce described the *formation* of a hypothesis as 'an act of insight', the 'abductive suggestion' coming to us 'like a flash' (cited in Sebeok and Umiker-Sebeok, 1983: 18). Abduction, for Peirce, is the first step of scientific reasoning, an instinct which relies upon unconscious perception of connections between aspects of the world, or to use another set of terms, subliminal communication of messages.

Eco outlines the difference between deduction and induction using an account from C.S. Peirce:

> I once landed at a seaport in a Turkish province; and as I was walking up to the house which I was to visit, I met a man upon horseback, surrounded by four horsemen holding a canopy over his head. As the governor of the province was the only personage I could think of who would be so greatly honored, I inferred that this was he. This was an hypothesis. (cited in Eco, 1983: 219)

Eco says that C.S. Peirce made two inferences. The first one was a hypothesis or deduction – he knew the general rule according to which a man with a canopy over his head, in Turkey, could not be anybody but an authority, and imagined that the man he met represented a case of that unquestionable rule. The second one was an inductive inference: of the various authorities that could have been in that place (why not a visiting minister from Istanbul?), the governor of the province was the most plausible.

The importance of the role of different styles of reasoning is often explicitly highlighted in detective fiction. In G.K. Chesterton's *The Blue Cross* (1987) the great French police detective Valentin is trying to track down Flambeau, a brilliant crook who, disguised as a priest, is travelling with Father Brown and planning to steal a valuable cross from him. Valentin resorted to guessing – abduction – when traditional 'logic' did not appear to be appropriate.

> Exactly because Valentin understood reason, he understood the limits of reason. Only a man who knows nothing of motors talks of a motoring without petrol; only a man who knows nothing of reason talks of reasoning without strong, undisputed first principles. Here he had no strong first principles. Flambeau had been missed at Harwich; and if he was in London at all, he might be anything from a tall tramp on Wimbledon Common to a tall toastmaster at the Hotel Metropole. In such a naked state of nescience, Valentin had a view and a method of his own.
>
> In such cases he reckoned on the unforeseen. In such cases, when he could not follow the train of the reasonable, he coldly and carefully followed the train of the unreasonable. Instead of going to the right places – banks, police-stations, rendezvous – he systematically went to the wrong places; knocked at every empty house, turned down every cul de sac, went up every lane blocked with rubbish, went round every crescent that had him uselessly out of the way. He defended this crazy course quite logically. He said that if one had a clue this was the worst way; but if one had no clue at all it was the best, because there was just the chance that any oddity that caught the eye of the pursuer might be the same that had caught the eye of the pursued.
>
> (Used by permission)

Father Brown, knowing Valentin's style of reasoning, leaves odd clues for Valentin to see, assuming that Valentin will observe things that do not obviously look like clues. Valentin's following of the 'train of the unreasonable' is not unlike Holmes's concern with 'trifles'.

Understanding the differences between deduction, induction and abduction is important to social science research and to quantitative methods. It allows researchers to understand the nature of the evidence that they are dealing with and the nature of the inferences that are being made about observations. Let's look a bit more closely at what is involved in the three different types of logical thinking. Traditional deductive reasoning is syllogistic.

For example,

All serious wounds lead to bleeding = All cases of serious wounding are cases of bleeding
This is a (case of) serious wounding
Therefore there is (this is a case of) bleeding

is an example of a valid syllogism.

C.S. Pierce and Umberto Eco, however, have an interest in possibilities and probabilities, and not in strict deductive reasoning. Inductive logic has an interest in judgements about individual cases and the build-up of evidence.

For example,

This is a (case of) serious wounding
This is (a case of) bleeding
Therefore perhaps (it is possible that) all serious wounds lead to bleeding

is a form of inductive reasoning.

With the statement above, you could also assert 'it is probable that' as a conclusion. This would be directly statistical, and could not be supported by one case alone.

In Peirce's abduction, we would need to introduce a further premise drawing or asserting a plausible connection in theory or observation, and we would get as a conclusion not assertion of fact but a hypothesis which would need independent testing.

Deduction in traditional logical reasoning does not involve wild guesses or flashes of insight – the conclusion must follow from the evidence; the fact under consideration can be inferred from certain other facts by means of specified general laws. The conclusion in the example of induction on the other hand is the most plausible explanation, given the evidence. Abductions, like inductions, are not logically self-contained, as is the deduction, and they need to be externally validated. The conclusion in the abduction represents a conjecture about reality which needs to be validated through testing.

Scientists quantify their observations in deductive and inductive styles of reasoning. Hempel gives a good example where a scientific explanation is inductive and where statistics are applied to assist with decision-making.

When Johnny comes down with the measles, this might be explained by pointing out that he caught the disease from his sister, who is just recovering from it. The particular antecedent facts here invoked are that of Johnny's exposure and, let us assume, the further fact that Johnny had not had the measles previously. But to connect these with the event to be explained, we cannot adduce a general law to the effect that under the specified circumstances, the measles is invariably transmitted to the exposed person: what can be asserted is only a high probability (in the sense of a statistical frequency) of transmission. The same type of argument can be used also for predicting or postdicting the occurrence of a case of the measles. (Hempel, 1965: 175)

In this example, statements about the cause of Johnny's measles take *statistical form*, giving a probability of transmission. There is no 'general law' that says measles is 'invariably transmitted' to the exposed person. The relationship between cause and effect does not take *universal form*.

Science and social science have in common the different styles of reasoning – at least superficially. Deduction, induction and abduction are quantitative. They include or exclude meanings and include or exclude particular conclusions. Evidence 'adds up'. Even guessing involves choices that include or exclude one kind of evidence over another. But can we simply translate notions of quantity and of measurement from science to social science? Logic might underpin both science and social science, but it is not clear that the phenomena of social science involve a simple correspondence between the measure and the phenomenon.

Causality

We do not know whether 19th century social theorists such as Emile Durkheim, August Comte or Herbert Spencer were, like Holmes, cocaine addicts. But like Holmes they did attempt to define their research in terms of the principles of the *science* of the day.

> Sociological explanation consists exclusively in establishing relationships of causality, that a phenomenon must be joined to its cause, or, on the contrary a cause to its useful effects. (Durkheim, 1964)

The implication here is that all reasoning in social science research is deductive and that all facts can be referred back to general laws. But, as we have seen, there are different styles of reasoning in detective fiction and not all our thinking or our conclusions are necessarily referable to general laws. Detectives, social scientists and ordinary human beings are often 'meta-betters', taking punts on knowledge and predicting what is going to happen in everyday life without full knowledge about the possible consequences.

Durkheim, however, has a point about 'establishing relationships'. Holmes in his analysis of Watson's thoughts is trying to establish a relationship between what he sees and what he knows about Watson and what Watson is, in fact, thinking. But Holmes cannot confirm his ideas of cause and effect until he talks to Watson. Much of quantitative social science research is about modelling relationships – finding out how phenomena are related – before causation is established.

Textbooks often make a distinction between **necessary** and **sufficient** causes. A necessary cause is a precondition without which a certain consequence will *not* come about, but which does not guarantee that this consequence *will* come about. A sufficient cause *does* guarantee the consequence. For example, a mixture of violently inflammable gases is a necessary cause for a gas explosion but not a sufficient one, or we would have more of them; setting a light to such a mixture, by contrast, is a sufficient cause. Becoming a Catholic monk is a sufficient cause for getting a habit; being a man is a necessary but not sufficient cause for becoming a monk. The distinction between 'necessary' and 'sufficient' causes can be fuzzy because what is 'necessary' and what is 'sufficient' may sometimes be a matter of point of view.

Trying to isolate causes is, of course, basic to detective fiction. Ellery Queen's novels provide readers with all the clues needed to solve the crime. It is up to the reader to try to establish the relationships between the clues and to deduce the cause of the crime (the killer or killers). 'By the exercise of strict logic and irrefutable deductions from given data, it should be simple for the reader to name at this point the murderer of Abigail Doorn and Dr. Francis Jannery. I say simple advisedly. Actually it is not simple; the deductions are natural, but they require sharp and unflagging thought' (Queen, 1983: 199).

The quantitative social scientist, however, is often in the position where he or she is trying to establish relationships but not trying (or not able) to establish causation. Correlation and causation are not the same in quantitative research methods. The reader of Ellery Queen's novels, for example, may come up with a statement of relationships between clues (correlation) but get the answer to the identity of the killer (causation) completely wrong – even though some of the reader's suggested relationships between clues are, in fact, correct.

Establishing relationships and establishing causation can be different. In defining our inquiry therefore it is worthwhile trying to 'map' our thoughts about the possible relationships between different phenomena that we observe. Sometimes it is worthwhile doing this graphically to check the logic of the relationships between phenomena.

Mapping Relationships

Turning a verbal statement into a diagram can be a useful first step in defining our research. Here are two paragraphs from Pugh and Hickson (1989: 115) with the points numbered for the diagram following:

> Innovative firms have an 'integrative' approach to problems. They have a willingness to see problems as wholes (1) and in their solutions to move beyond received wisdom (2), to challenge established practices. Entrepreneurial organisations [in this context just another way of saying 'innovative organisations'] are willing to operate at the edges of their competence, dealing with what they do not yet know (2 repeated). - - -
>
> They contrast very strongly with firms with a 'segmentalist' approach. These see problems as narrowly as possible, independently of their context. Companies like this are likely to have segmented structures (3); a large number of compartments strongly walled off from one another – production department from marketing department, corporate managers from divisional managers, management from labour, men from women. As soon as a problem is identified it is broken up and the parts dealt with by the appropriate departments. Little or no effort is given to the problem as an integrated whole. – So entrepreneurial spirit is stifled and the solution is unlikely to be innovative.

41

All the words in these sentences create a meaningful picture of organizations – especially the second kind. But a diagram puts it more succinctly. Here is the diagram drawn from the numbers in the sentences:

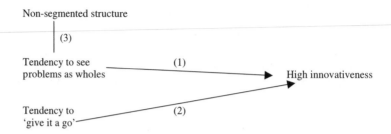

Changing 'move beyond received wisdom and operate at the edges of competence' to the Australianism 'give it a go' is a free translation. There is no arrow-head on (3) because arrows go from cause to effect – or more properly from **independent** to **dependent variables** of a pair – and in this case the author does not tell us which causes which. Sociological common sense suggests that it should be a double arrow or one with points on both ends because each will maintain and enhance the other in a vicious circle, but this is diagramming two paragraphs and they do not say this themselves.

When we are linking **variables** common sense will usually tell us which way the arrows go, but there are rules of thumb. Here is a list of rules, from Harvard Sociology's Davis of the 'Davis d' (Davis, 1985: 11–16)

1   'Run the arrow from X to Y if Y starts after X freezes.' Run an arrow from (e.g.) childhood schooling pointing to adult income but not the other way round, because childhood schooling is over before adult income starts and nothing outside of science fiction can change the past.
2   'Run the arrow from X to Y if X is linked to an earlier step in a well-known sequence'; this is merely an extension of the first rule, for when X did not actually stop happening ('freeze') before Y started, but it still came first in a sequence of events.
3   'Run the arrow from X to Y if X never changes and Y sometimes changes'; thus never put *sex* (for example) at the pointed end of the arrow – sex can cause all sorts of things, but nothing in the world can cause widespread sex-changes. Birth year, race, and national origin work the same way.
4   'Run the arrow from X to Y if X is more stable, harder to change, or more fertile'; a 'fertile' event or quality is one well known to have a lot of effects, like being married or not or living in this or that neighbourhood. Davis lists some other contrasts between the 'relatively sticky' and 'relatively loose' attributes, the former probable causes and the latter probable effects. Here is part of it; note that the left and right concepts on the one line are not juxtaposed – it is just two lists:

Relatively sticky	*Relatively loose*
religious preference	presidential popularity
occupational prestige	happiness, morale
household composition	stands on political issues
political party identification	media habits
Intelligence Quotient	preferences for candidates (or brands)

Now let's go to another and more complicated causal diagram, again start-
ing with the statement as read: This passage is from an article in *Higher
Education Research & Development* (1984: 66) reporting a study of Australian
National University students:

> Of the independent variables, age was found to be the best predictor of academic
> performance in Behavioural Science students (1). [This] could be explained, first,
> by their higher motivation and determination to succeed in their study as
> compared to younger age students (2). As evidence of this, many researchers
> (e.g. Boon, 1980) have reported these students as having few motivational prob-
> lems (2 again) and as being conscientious and hard working in their approaches
> towards study (3). The fact that older age students undertaking tertiary study
> generally enter self-selected courses (4), and are most willing to make consider-
> able personal sacrifices (5) may well explain their high motivation and determina-
> tion. Secondly, older age students on the whole have the distinct advantage (6) of
> accumulated knowledge and experience (6) due to maturity, referred to by Knox
> (1977) as 'crystallized intelligence', which would enhance their academic perform-
> ance (7), and be useful particularly in the study of Behavioural Science. Thirdly, a
> large proportion of older age students undertake their studies on a part-time basis
> (8). The observed difference in the academic performance of these students may
> be a function of their different attendance patterns. There is considerable evidence
> of part-time students performing better than full-time students (9) (e.g. Butterfield
> & Kane, 1969).

Let us look at a possible diagram:

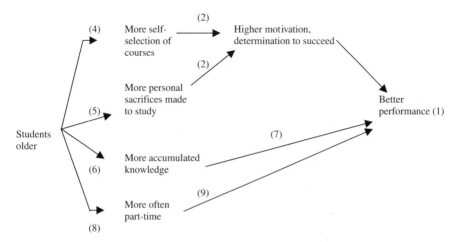

We have not run an arrow for (1) directly from 'older students' to 'better performance' because the argument purports to explain all this in terms of the other variables. The statement (3) has no arrow because it relates to a statement of *evidence* for causation rather than of causation as such.

The arrow from 'motivation/determination to succeed' to 'better performance' has no number because the argument does not actually say that the two factors are positively linked. This is unlike (7) and (8) where we are told and given references for the ideas that 'accumulated knowledge' and 'being a part-timer' in fact goes with better performance.

Sherlock Holmes talks in the language of 'cause and effect'. It is possible, as Umberto Eco says, to conceptually map Holmes's arguments of 'causation' and to decide where Holmes is guessing and where he is not; where the evidence for the links between cause and effect are clear and where they are not. In social science research it is also possible to conceptually map causal relationships, even if we have not measured these relationships. In the diagramming above we have briefly raised the idea of relationships between phenomena – hypothesizing relationships and independent and dependent variables, what Holmes might call his 'trifles'. Let's now examine these trifles in more detail.

TOOLS OF MEASUREMENT

'AM CROSSING TO GET MEXICAN DIVORCE STOP WILL MARRY CHRIS STOP GOOD LUCK AND GOODBYE CRYSTAL' (Chandler, 1944: 18)

This is a telegram Derace Kingsley received from his wife. Kingsley knew that his wife was having affairs but doubted the truth of the note. He employed Phillip Marlowe, Chandler's famous seedy detective, to track down the truth. Marlowe goes through a detailed discussion with Kingsley to find out the context of Crystal's disappearance. Marlowe, in this story, has ideas about the relationships between events associated with Crystal's disappearance and, as the story unfolds, the causes of her disappearance.

Hypotheses in detective fiction are statements about the relationships between possible facts or observations. In the social sciences we also have hypotheses as statements of possible facts. These statements normally go through a process of operationalization – procedures for classifying, ordering and measuring variables. In social science research there are two major types of measurable hypotheses – correlational and causal.

Correlational statements take the form:

'Is there a relationship between X and Y?'

Correlational hypotheses test a hypothesis about two or more variables by measuring the variables to see if they are related. The statement 'People with unstable marriages are more likely to have atheistic upbringings' would be a correlational hypothesis. It is not a hypothesis where you could properly manipulate a variable – require people to have a particular type of upbringing for the sake of a study – or say that one variable depends on another.

Causal statements take the form:

'If you manipulate the independent variable I, then you will observe a change in the dependent variable D'.

Correlational hypotheses can be 'causal', but the independent variable is not (or cannot be) manipulated. Experiments are often associated with the *Experimenters link* more traditional causal hypotheses. Experimenters try to vary the independent variable(s) and account in a controlled way for other variables that might be mistaken for causes. The word 'make' in a sentence suggests a causal hypothesis. 'A private education makes people more tolerant of extra-marital sexual behaviour' would be a causal statement. But could we manipulate the independent variable? Could we ethically change a person's potential education to see what the effects would be?

Criteria for good hypotheses are logical and not mathematical. Hypotheses must be:

1 consistent with current knowledge;
2 logically consistent (if a hypothesis suggests that $A = B$ and $B = C$, then A must also be equal to C); if reading The London Times implies a knowledge of current affairs, and a knowledge of current events means greater participation in social activities, then readers should exhibit greater participation in social activities;
3 parsimonious (the simpler the better);
4 testable and/or realistic.

One of the most difficult tasks for the social scientist is to define the constructs and variables within the study and the hypothesis. The definition and measurement of variables are intimately linked.

What are Variables?

In the social sciences we assume that attributes of a phenomenon are measurable – male and female are, for example, attributes of 'sex'. When we say something is measurable then we are saying that attributes possess a structure that is quantitative and therefore quantifiable. In what sense are these attributes measurable? The most commonly used definition of measurement in the social sciences is the one formulated by Stevens (1946). He said that measurement is the assignment of numbers to objects or events

45

according to rules. We assign numbers to attributes in such a way that the properties of the attributes are faithfully represented by the properties of the numbers. Variables are, therefore, the embodiment of both constructs that we want to define and the numbers that we use to represent them.

A variable is a general class of objects, events, situations, characteristics and attributes that are of interest to the researcher. In the social sciences we are usually interested in variables to do with people. The psychologist, for example, is interested in behavioural or psychological variables such as cognitive ability, personality and psychophysiological reactions, such as stress. The main feature of a variable is that it can have different values. Your age may be different from that of your best friend, your income may be different from your best friend's income. The values a variable can take on vary. Importantly, these attributes or variables are measurable.

We do not investigate variables in isolation. The basic aim of any quantitative research is to investigate how variables interact with each other. Some investigations simply look at how variables co-relate. But on other occasions, we might ask more specific research questions about the nature of these relationships. We might, for example, ask whether one variable X (say, amount of time spent studying for an exam) influences another variable Y (final mark on that exam). As mentioned in the brief discussion on causal hypotheses, we refer to variable X as the *independent variable* and Y as the *dependent variable*. The independent variable has an impact on the dependent variable. In other words, the values that the dependent variable takes on are influenced by the independent variable. The relationship may not necessarily be causal, because the ability of the student may also influence his or her final exam mark, not just the amount of time spent studying. Be careful therefore of causal imagery inherent in this relationship.

Variables can be operationalized at various levels of measurement. Stevens (1951) distinguished four levels of quantification or measurement – nominal, ordinal, interval and ratio measurement. *Nominal or categorical* – level measurement consists of unordered categories. Each category can be given a name or a number. For example, the variable 'gender' has two categories or levels, male and female. We can use the words 'male' and 'female' to identify people that belong to each category or we can assign numbers to each category such that the number represents that category. For instance, the number 1 may be assigned to represent 'females' and the number 2 to represent 'males'. This level of measurement allows us to assess whether people are from the same or a different category.

Ordinal-level measurement has the properties of nominal scales with the additional property that the categories can be rank-ordered. If the categories of a variable are ordered, that is, category B has 'more' of the phenomenon being measured than category A, then we say that that variable can be measured on an ordinal scale. We assign numbers to each category such that the ordering property inherent in the variable is preserved by the numbers or scores assigned. For instance, if John is taller than Bill, we can assign the number 2 to John and 1 to Bill. The number 2 is greater than 1, so the relationship between these two numbers preserves the height relationship between John and Bill. The property then allows us to rank-order the values of variables measured on ordinal scales. These ranks can then be validly compared.

Interval-level measurement has the defining property that equal intervals on a scale represent equal amounts of the quantity being measured. If we are measuring income in dollars, then the difference between annual incomes of $45,000 and $50,000 is the same amount as the difference between someone who earns $55,000 and someone who earns $60,000. That is to say, there is a difference of $5,000 and that difference is 'the same' (representing the same monetary value) for each comparison of incomes. Similarly, assume you are asked to rate the content of three television programmes in terms of humour using a five-point scale where '0' means 'not at all funny' and '4' means 'extremely funny'. If we can demonstrate that the difference (in terms of the amount of humour represented in the variable) in ratings between '0' and '1' is the same as the difference between ratings of '3' and '4', then we are using an interval scale. Clearly, establishing this property in this case may be difficult. As Watson et al. (1993: 38) noted, 'It is possible to specify, to some degree, what properties the observations should have in order to lead to interval scale measurement and then to investigate whether these properties are actually met by the observations'. Cliff (1996) argues on the other hand that in the social sciences we can only achieve ordinal-level measurement.

A fourth level of measurement, *ratio-level* measurement, has all the properties of ordinal and interval measurement. However, ratio measurement has the additional property that equal ratios between numbers on the scale represent equal ratios of the attribute being measured. Height measured in centimetres (cm) is an example of ratio measurement. Someone who is 180 cm tall is twice the height of someone who is 90 cm tall. Similarly, weight measured in kilograms (kg) is a ratio measure. A person who is 120 kg is twice the weight of someone who is 60 kg; someone weighing 90 kg is twice the weight of someone weighing 45 kg. An additional property of ratio measurement is that there is a zero point on the scale that indicates the absence of the attribute being measured. The examples of weight measured in kilograms and height measured in centimetres both have a zero scale (i.e. 0 kg or 0 cm) value that indicates the absence of either weight or height.

It is difficult to establish whether many types of measures in the social sciences are in fact interval- and ratio-level measurement. The fact that many texts, including this one, use natural science examples to show how interval and ratio scales work is itself an indication. Indeed many researchers argue that there are relatively few examples of ratio-level measurement in the social sciences. Are there other ways of classifying or describing data obtained from variables? Data may be referred to as *qualitative* when the scale used for measuring that variable is a set of unordered categories, that is, the level of measurement is nominal. In this case the categories are *qualitatively* different; they do not vary in magnitude or *quantity*. Nominal measures are often called *discrete variables* because they cannot be subdivided. Means and medians are not normally calculated for discrete variables. When data from variables vary in magnitude, they are referred to as *quantitative* data. Variables measured on interval or ratio scales can be described as quantitative. Interval and ratio measures are often called *continuous variables* because they can be subdivided. The nature of ordinal data is a little fuzzy. Ordinal scales consist of categories, therefore they can be thought of as qualitative. Ordinal scales also have categories that are greater than or less than each other in magnitude and are therefore quantitative. Ordinal scales, however, are normally treated as discrete variables (Agresti and Findlay, 1997).

Operational Definitions

The levels of measurement represent the mathematical possibilities available to you for quantitative analysis – such as adding, subtracting, multiplying and dividing – when you have decided how you want to define the phenomenon you want to study; how to measure your observations. Definition, however, precedes measurement. Some phenomena are easier to define and to measure than others. For example, sex, already mentioned, can be measured with the values 1 representing 'female' and 2 representing 'male'. But you cannot subtract 'male' from 'female' or divide them!

If I say that I want to operationalize 'gender' as a nominal variable, I am unlikely to encounter great debate. But not all constructs or phenomena are that easy to measure or that easy to get an agreement on. This is not surprising – in social science most if not all phenomena that we wish to study come from everyday life or from phenomena that are not easily observable. We use language to describe and to define the phenomena that we wish to measure. We try to measure constructs described by language that we hope corresponds to the phenomenon of interest. Figure 3.1 summarizes the steps in measurement.

Your 'construct' is your idea about the phenomenon that you want to measure. Your operational definition is your statement about how you want to measure your construct. The construct 'deliquency', for example, might be operationally defined by 'being arrested more than once prior to the age

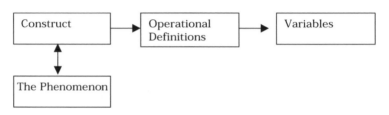

FIGURE 3.1 *Operationalization*

18'. In a questionnaire you might have the question (your variable) 'Have you been arrested more than once prior to the age 18? Yes. No.' This is a nominal-level question. *This is one variable.* It is also possible to imagine other definitions and operational definitions of the construct that might be useful.

Defining and measuring our observations in social science can be affected by the society that we live in. For example, *The Information Bulletin of the Reich Association of Aryan Christians* in Nazi Germany sought to quantify Aryanism – the idea that blonde blue-eyed people are superior to everyone else – in order to reduce uncertainty among Christians about who and who was not a Jew. The Association provided Christians with definitions of what constituted 'Aryan':

> Question: A man has two Jewish grandparents, one Aryan grandmother and a half-Aryan grandfather; the latter was born Jewish and became Christian only later. Is this 62 percent Jewish person a Mischling or a Jew?

> Answer: The man is a Jew according to the Nuremburg Laws because of the one grandparent who was of the Jewish religion; this grandparent is assumed to have been a full Jew and this assumption cannot be contested. So this 62 percent Jew has three full Jewish grandparents. On the other hand, if the half-Aryan grandfather had been Christian by birth, he would not then have been a full Jew and would not have counted at all for this calculation; his grandson would have been a Mischling of the First Degree. (Friedlander, 1997: 158)

Such statements are, for all intents and purposes, 'operational definitions'. They are quantifications. But they are quantifications based on inferences about observations that are biased by society. Moreover, the definitions themselves have social consequences. Being a Mischling meant survival, of course. Mischling were treated better than full Jews. The construct 'Jew', therefore, was not a neutral category, nor was it a 'natural' phenomenon.

Let us take another example from a well-known scholar.

> The Jew, who is something of a nomad, has never yet created a cultural form of his own and as far as we can see never will, since all his instincts and talents require a more or less civilized nation to act as a host for their development.... The Aryan consciousness has a higher potential than the Jewish; that is both the advantage and the disadvantage of a youthfulness not yet fully weaned from barbarism. (1997: 171)

No. This is not a statement from Adolf Hitler or Joseph Goebbels. It is Carl Jung, the famous psychoanalyst, in 1934 singing the praises of National Socialist Nazi Germany. Can we infer from Jung's statement that he is an anti-semite? Is Jung, at base, no different from other Nazis? Jung belongs to the same style of reasoning about Jewishness. He uses the same *language* as everyone else in Nazi Germany. He does not need the fear of the

Gestapo (barely formed in 1934) to come up with his ideas about Aryan civilization.

Nazi German scientists, psychologists and psychiatrists were committed to the idea of Aryan superiority and Jewish inferiority and tried to measure these constructs as if they were natural phenomena. Such 'measures', of course, have little to do with science and 'natural phenomena' and a lot to do with extreme and dangerous prejudice. The example highlights the problem with measurement in social science. Prejudice is the real phenomenon of interest in the example from Nazi Germany. 'Deductions' about Aryanism made by Nazi Germans of good will, though, show that styles of reasoning – deduction, induction and abduction – are not necessarily 'neutral' forms of reasoning. There were deductive premises associated with 'Jewishness' in the minds of Nazis. Observations were used to reinforce those premises as if there were a universal law about Aryanism and Jewishness. The authors have called deduction, induction and abduction 'styles of reasoning', following Ian Hacking's (1982) phrase, precisely because those styles may be subordinated to the ideology of the day.

Contemporary Views on Measurement

In his account of Dr Watson's thoughts Sherlock Holmes said he was being deductive when he was, in fact, guessing. In social science we deal with constructs and try to provide measures for these constructs. For example, we assume that a measurement of the construct 'self-esteem' is also a measurement of the phenomenon 'self-esteem'. We are, in some senses, 'meta-betting', even at this stage. As you have seen, we have to be very careful. Does the measurement of the construct really measure the under-lying phenomenon?

Recall that Stevens' definition of measurement involves the application of a set of rules for assigning numbers to objects, people, attributes and so on. In recent times, this definition of measurement has been questioned inside and outside of statistics. Michell (1997, 1999) argues that there is a discrepancy between a traditional understanding of measurement in the natural sciences and the Stevens definition of measurement. The traditional view of measurement is the discovery of real numerical relations (ratios) between things (magnitudes of attributes), and not the attempt to construct conventional numerical relations where they do not otherwise exist (Michell, 1999: 17). Michell illustrates this point as follows:

> In measurement, according to the traditional view, numbers (or numerals) are not assigned to anything. If, for example, I discover by measuring it that my room is 4 metres long, neither the number four nor the numeral 4 is assigned to anything, any more than if I observe that the wall of my room is red, either the colour red or the word *red* is thereby assigned to anything. In neither case am I dealing with the assignment of one thing to another. Considering the ratios of magnitudes and

the numbers involved in measurement, it is clear that one is not dealing with the relation of assignment. One is dealing, rather, with predication. That is, it is not that my room or its length is related to the number four, the length of my room relative to the metre simply is the number four.' (1999: 17)

Michell says that quantitative science involves two tasks, namely (1) investigating that the attribute of interest is in fact quantitative, and (2) devising procedures to measure the magnitude of quantitative attributes. In the social sciences, and especially psychology, researchers have assumed that variables are quantitative. We assume, for example, that psychological variables such as self-esteem and extroversion are by their nature quantitative. For Michell (1997), though, phenomena like self-esteem have no clear unit of measurement compared with a cricket pitch where the measure of the pitch is related to the pitch.

This sounds a warning to us about the nature of measurement in the social sciences, but it is not a warning to reject measurement altogether. Let's investigate a theorist who attempted to measure a complex phenomenon – how cultures vary. Geert Hofstede applies a contemporary view of measurement. He knows that he is measuring constructs. He is also aware that there are issues associated with the relationship between the definitions of a construct and its measurement.

GREAT SOCIOLOGICAL DETECTIVE STORIES: Collecting Data Across Cultures: Can we measure cultural variation? *Culture's Consequences* (Geert Hofstede)

Geert Hofstede is a sociological detective who worked on a global scale. He raised questions about the problems associated with the creation of a world culture before globalization, personal computers and the internet became trendy in the study of intercultural communication. Hofstede wanted to quantify how cultures vary and why. He conducted surveys in 66 countries within subsidiaries of a large multinational business. He ran the pioneer international surveys twice, in 1968 and 1972, producing a total of over 116,000 questionnaires.

The origin of Hofstede's major study was a multinational company's concern with employee morale. HERMES, the cover name Hosftede gave to the multinational company to protect its identity, was a service company that had employees and customers located throughout the world. An important part of the corporate philosophy was that customer satisfaction and employee morale were related. Employee attitude surveys fitted well in this context. Hofstede headed a team to prepare the first internationally standardized questionnaire for the simultaneous survey of the corporation's personnel.

Methodology and Theory

In order to study corporate morale on an international scale Hofstede developed a methodology that enabled him to measure employee attitudes in different cultural contexts. He did not have at hand a simple methodology to assist him. Methodology is 'the science of finding out' (Babbie, 1986: 6). It is the philosophical and theoretical underpinning of research that affects what a researcher counts as evidence. Methods are the actual techniques, like Hofstede's international questionnaires, and procedures used to quantify and to collect data. While 'methodology' and 'methods' are different conceptually they are of course related. Methodology affects method choice. When Sherlock Holmes told Dr Watson 'you know my method', he was combining in this phrase both his assumption about law-like behaviour and the actual techniques of deduction that he said he used. The distinction between 'nomothetic' and 'idiographic', raised briefly in Chapters 1 and 2, relates to theory and methodology. Nomothetic and idiographic represent different styles of inquiry. Understanding society 'from the inside' and through definitions of its members has been called ethnoscience, ethnography or ethnomethodology (among others). Understanding society 'from the outside', by the creation of general classifications or general laws of behaviour, has been called functionalism, positivism or empiricism (among others). Hofstede was faced with a difficulty. An 'idiographic' approach would assume that each culture is unique and no one law or classification can govern them all. A 'nomothetic' approach would suggest there are comparisons that can be made across cultures and values that affect all cultures. 'The pure idiographer will probably shy away from quantitative data and the use of statistics. Those collecting comparative data that lend themselves to statistical analysis will be attracted to different statistical methods according to their degree of nomotheticity' (Hofstede, 1984: 33).

Detectives in detection fiction also have their 'degree of nomotheticity'. Some detectives try to see whether there is a typical kind of behaviour (called 'ideal types' in sociology), and back it up with examples. This is idiographic (and inductive, of course). Other detectives assume 'law-like theories' that enable them to predict what is going to happen. This is nomothetic. Dr Spock in the science fiction *Star Trek* is presented as a cold, calculating, character who thinks only logically and scientifically (rather than emotionally). This is, perhaps, like Sherlock Holmes, the stereotype of the 'nomothetic' model.

Hofstede decided to take a middle road – combining the specific and the general. His theory was based on the idea of 'mental programmes'. Each person, group and culture, says Hofstede, carries a certain amount of mental programming which is stable over time. He says that in everyday life we often use constructs to describe these mental programmes – for example 'all members of the family will come if I ring the dinner bell'. The task for Hofstede therefore was to look for measures of the constructs that describe mental programmes associated with cultural values – 'to find observable phenomena from which the construct can be inferred' (1984: 17).

Method

Hypotheses and Operationalization

Hoftstede's theoretical hypothesis is that cultural values – specific quantifiable dimensions of cultural value – have consequences for organizational behaviour (and for human behaviour generally) and the 'mental programmes' associated with this behaviour. 'As nearly all our mental programs are affected by values, nearly all are affected by culture, and this is reflected by our behaviours' (1984: 23). Hofstede defined 'values' as 'a broad tendency to prefer certain states of affairs over others' (1984: 18). Cultural values are 'independent variables' for Hofstede and a diagram would look something like this:

Cultural values ⟶ Structure and functioning of institutions (e.g. education, religion)

Hofstede's literature review covered cross-cultural or cross-national studies from the disciplines of psychology (cross-cultural psychology), sociology (organizational psychology), anthropology, political science, economics, geography, history, comparative law, comparative medicine and international market research.

Hoftstede identified from his literature review and preliminary analyses (he of course pre-tested his questionnaires) what he thought were four major dimensions of cultural value – individualism, power distance, uncertainty avoidance and masculinity. He created 60 core questions, 60 variables, for his questionnaire which clustered in four main areas.

1 Satisfactions – 'supply a personal evaluation of an aspect of the work situation – 'How satisfied are you with ...' but also 'How do you like your job – the kind of work you do?'
2 Perceptions – subjective descriptions of an aspect or problem of the work situation – 'How often does your manager expect a large amount of work from you?'
3 Personal goals and belief – statements not about the job or the company as such but related to an ideal job or to general issues in industry – for example 'How important is it to you to have an opportunity for high earnings?'
4 Demographics – age, sex, years of education, years with the company, and so on.

Table 3.1 gives a brief overview of Hoftstede's process of operationalization.

TABLE 3.1   *From construct to operational definition*

Construct	Defined as	Operationally defined by
Cultural values	'a broad tendency to prefer certain states of affairs over others' (1984: 18)	Scores/indexes for individualism, uncertainty avoidance, power distance, masculinity

TABLE 3.2   *Actual questions used to construct individualism/masculinity indexes*

Challenge – Have challenging work to do – work from which you can get a personal sense of accomplishment
Desirable area – Live in an area desirable to you and your family
Earnings – Have an opportunity for high earnings
Cooperation – Work with people who cooperate well with one another
Training – Have training opportunities (to improve your skills or learn new skills)
Benefits – Have good fringe benefits
Recognition – Get the recognition you deserve when you do a good job
Physical conditions – Have good physical working conditions (good ventilation and lighting, adequate work space, etc)
Freedom – Have considerable freedom to adapt your own approach to the job
Employment security – Have the security that you will be able to work for your company as long as you want to
Advancement – Have an opportunity for advancement to higher level jobs
Manager – Have a good working relationship with your manager
Use of skills – Fully use your skills and abilities on the job
Personal time – Have a job which leaves you sufficient time for your personal or family life

Source: (1984: 155)

Let's look at how Hofstede went about constructing the dimensions of culture, the 'cultural values', from his variables. Two of his major dimensions, individualism and masculinity, were derived from the questions in Table 3.2. These questions, which were prefaced with 'How important is it to you to...', were designed to cover key issues such as desire for, say, a sense of freedom (which would be related to individualism) and desire for greater earnings (masculinity).

A man might, of course, provide answers that would be classified in the 'feminine' dimension. On the masculinity dimension, Hofstede confirmed previous findings on gender differences – that there are significant differences in responses from men and women:

More important for men:

Advancement
Earnings
Training
Up-to-datedness

More important for women:

Friendly atmosphere
Position security
Physical conditions

Manager
Cooperation

Hofstede's sociology is an ambitious attempt to bridge the 'idiographic' – the individual motivations and desires of individuals in their local situation – with the 'nomothetic' – the general causes and general classifications – cultural values – that affect those individuals and those situations. The results of Hofstede's analysis included a detailed ranking of countries by the different dimensions of culture.

Variables

A more detailed examination of the results of Hoftstede's study provides a better sense of what he was trying to achieve with the major dimensions of culture.

Individualism and Masculinity

In individualistic countries (like the US, Australia, UK) people's personal goals take priority over their allegiance to groups like the family or the employer. Competition rather than cooperation is encouraged; personal goals take precedence over group goals; people tend not to be emotionally dependent on organizations and institutions; and every individual has the right to his or her thoughts and opinions. These cultures emphasize individual initiative and achievement and they value decision-making.

In collective societies (like Pakistan, Taiwan, Peru) people are born into extended families or clans that support and protect them in exchange for their loyalty. Identity is based on the social system; the individual is emotionally dependent on organizations and institutions; the culture emphasizes belonging to organizations; organizations invade private life and the clans to which individuals belong; and individuals trust group decisions. According to Hofstede, for example, the Japanese value collectivism over individualism, collaboration over competition.

Hofstede ranked countries on an individualism/collectivism scale. A high score means the country can be classified as collective. A lower score is associated with cultures that can be classified as individualistic. Table 3.3 presents the rankings on individualism.

Countries were also be ranked by 'masculine' and 'feminine' traits. Masculinity, for Hofstede, is the extent to which dominant values within a society are male-oriented and are associated with such behaviours as assertiveness, ambition, achievement, the acquisition of money, signs of manliness, material possessions, and not caring for others. Ireland, for example, tends to masculinity, on Hofstede's scores. Femininity stresses caring and nurturing behaviour. Table 3.4 shows Hofstede's rankings on this dimension.

TABLE 3.3 *Countries ranked by individualism scores*

USA	1	India	21
Australia	2	Japan	22
Great Britain	3	Argentina	23
Canada	4	Iran	24
Netherlands	5	Brazil	25
New Zealand	6	Turkey	26
Italy	7	Greece	27
Belgium	8	Philippines	28
Denmark	9	Mexico	29
Sweden	10	Portugal	30
France	11	Yugoslavia	31
Ireland	12	Hong Kong	32
Norway	13	Chile	33
Switzerland	14	Singapore	34
Germany	15	Thailand	35
South Africa	16	Taiwan	36
Finland	17	Peru	37
Austria	18	Pakistan	38
Israel	19	Columbia	39
Spain	20	Venezuela	40

TABLE 3.4 *Countries ranked by masculinity scores*

Japan	1	Canada	21
Austria	2	Pakistan	22
Venezuela	3	Brazil	23
Italy	4	Singapore	24
Switzerland	5	Israel	25
Mexico	6	Turkey	26
Ireland	7	Taiwan	27
Great Britain	8	Iran	28
Germany	9	France	29
Philippines	10	Spain	30
Columbia	11	Peru	31
South Africa	12	Thailand	32
USA	13	Portugal	33
Australia	14	Chile	34
New Zealand	15	Finland	35
Greece	16	Yugoslavia	36
Hong Kong	17	Denmark	37
Argentina	18	Netherlands	38
India	19	Norway	39
Belgium	20	Sweden	40

Power Distance

One of the most important questions used to measure power distance was: 'How frequently, in your experience, does the following problem occur: employees being afraid to express disagreement with their managers?' Answers were provided on a five-point scale from very frequently to

TABLE 3.5   Countries ranked by power distance scores

Philippines	1	Pakistan	21
Mexico	2	Japan	22
Venezuela	3	Italy	23
India	4	South Africa	24
Yugoslavia	5	Argentina	25
Singapore	6	USA	26
Brazil	7	Canada	27
Hong Kong	8	Netherlands	28
France	9	Australia	29
Columbia	10	Germany	30
Turkey	11	Great Britain	31
Belgium	12	Switzerland	32
Peru	13	Finland	33
Thailand	14	Norway	34
Chile	15	Sweden	35
Portugal	16	Ireland	36
Greece	17	New Zealand	37
Iran	18	Denmark	38
Taiwan	19	Israel	39
Spain	20	Austria	40

very seldom. According to Hofstede, people in high power distance countries, such as India, Singapore and Greece, believe that power and authority are facts of life. These cultures instruct their members that people are not equal and that everybody has a rightful place. Children seldom interrupt the teacher and show great reverence and respect for authority. Low power distance countries, such as Austria, Finland and Denmark, hold that inequality in society should be minimized. People in these cultures believe they are close to power and should have access to that power. The rankings are presented in Table 3.5.

Uncertainty Avoidance

Two major questions were used in the measurement of uncertainty avoidance, one associated with rule orientation and one associated with employment stability. The rule orientation question was 'Company rules should not be broken – even if the employee thinks it is in the company's best interests' with the answer on a five-point scale from strongly agree to strongly disagree. The employment stability question was 'How long do you think you will continue working for this company?' with answers 2 years at the most, From 2 to 5 years, More than 5 years (but I probably will leave before I retire), Until I retire.

High uncertainty avoidance cultures try to avoid uncertainty and ambiguity by providing stability for their members – not tolerating deviant ideas and behaviours and believing in absolute truths. They are also characterized by a higher level of anxiety and stress: people think of the uncertainty inherent in life as a continuous hazard that must be avoided and there is a strong need for written rules (e.g. Portugal, Greece, Germany). Countries like Sweden and Denmark, however, prize initiative, and according to Hofstede are more willing to take risks, are more flexible and think that there should be as few rules as possible. The rankings for Sweden and Denmark are given in Table 3.6.

Hofstede took his indices of cultural difference to be tentative, subject to modification if additional empirical evidence came his way. Indeed, in Appendix 3 of his book *Culture's Consequences* he explicitly asks readers to send him information that might assist in his detective work: 'Please tell about examples from your own experience of differences in behaviour among people, groups, or institutions which differ in their nationalities but are otherwise comparable. Please mention the year and the place of your observations and the precise nationalities involved' (1984: 289). Hoftstede also asks readers to contact him if they had collected or discovered any measurements that might correlate with his indices of individualism, uncertainty avoidance, power distance or masculinity '(falsification is as important as verification!)' (1984: 289).

Hoftstede recognized that his own prejudices and values might shape his interpretation of the data – 'few human activities can be value free' (1984: 287). In Appendix 2 of *Culture's Consequences* he outlines his own values. Hoftstede's indices, however, show that he conceives of society as a system and that his idea of cultural values fits into the idea of a system. Social norms, value systems of major groups of population, have a regulating function. Social norms lead to the development and maintenance of institu-

TABLE 3.6 *Countries ranked by uncertainty avoidance scores*

Country	Rank	Country	Rank
Greece	1	Germany	21
Portugal	2	Thailand	22
Chile	3	Iran	23
Belgium	4	Finland	24
Japan	5	Switzerland	25
Yugoslavia	6	Netherlands	26
Peru	7	Australia	27
France	8	Norway	28
Spain	9	South Africa	29
Argentina	10	New Zealand	30
Turkey	11	Canada	31
Mexico	12	USA	32
Israel	13	Philippines	33
Columbia	14	India	34
Venezuela	15	Great Britain	35
Brazil	16	Ireland	36
Italy	17	Hong Kong	37
Pakistan	18	Sweden	38
Austria	19	Denmark	39
Taiwan	20	Singapore	40

tions (like the family) in society. It is possible to see the deductive (and causal) reasoning in Hoftstede's conceptual schema. He is more like a Sherlock Holmes than a Father Brown.

Hoftstede's work crosses business and academic domains. His is a good example of a study that was constructed to address practical business concerns (staff morale) and deeper theoretical issues (the nature of societies in different countries). Hoftstede's work is also a good example of the process of operationalization – going from constructs to description of those constructs to operational definition of those constructs.

SUMMARY

Human inquiry is a social activity. Research is a way of knowing. People are hypothesis testers even when they are not scientists. Deduction, induction, abduction (or retroduction) are the basic processes of reasoning in science and social science and represent different ways of testing ideas about the world around us, natural and social. Detectives in detective fiction are often stereotypical examples of these different styles of reasoning. Deduction is a process of reasoning that looks on the surface to be the most 'deterministic' – the conclusion must follow from the evidence. Induction is where the build-up of evidence is so great that the conclusion fits the facts. Abduction is the art of guessing, but guessing that still needs to be tested with evidence.

The different styles of reasoning show how the logic of inclusion and exclusion of evidence occurs. The process is, on the surface, quantitative, because it includes and excludes options. However, the example from Nazi Germany about attempts to quantify Aryanism shows that the styles of logical reasoning are not necessarily a protection from the effects of ideology and the system of beliefs within a society. The inferences from our observations may be directly affected by our beliefs about the phenomenon that we are studying. However, the public nature of social science – its openness to critique – is intended as a protection against abuse of research. Application of established codes of ethics is also intended as protection of human dignity. These codes will be revisited in later chapters.

The different styles of reasoning also raise traditional theoretical concerns about the relationship between the specific and the general; the 'idiographic' and the 'nomothetic'. Can we really measure the big picture? Holmes assumed that his observations of Watson's non-verbal behaviour were referable to general laws in a process of deduction. Holmes, however, guessed. It is easy to confuse the different styles of reasoning and to treat phenomena as law-like when they are, in fact, not.

Many of the statements that we make in social science are statements about relationships and statements about causation – is one thing related to another? has one thing affected another thing? The different styles of logical reasoning deal with statements of relationships between constructs. There is no shortage of people's statements about relationships, as we saw in the discussion on causal diagramming. However, we also found that mapping relationships is a complex business. We need to be careful that the phenomena that we are investigating are logically related. Watching television, for example, does not change you into a male or a female, but there may be differences between males and females in their viewing behaviour.

Statements about relationships between constructs are called hypotheses. Social scientists often want to measure these statements and these relationships. A statement of relationship between variables is an attempt to measure the underlying phenomena of interest to the researcher. Quantitative hypotheses can be correlational or causal. Correlational hypotheses investigate relationships that may or may not be causal, but there is no manipulation of the independent variable. Traditional causal hypotheses assume that the researcher is going to manipulate the independent variable. The independent variable is the assumed cause and the dependent variable is the assumed effect.

The process of definition and measurement of variables is called **operationalization.** There are four major levels of measurement for variables – nominal, ordinal, interval and ratio. Some variables, like income, can be operationalized at more than one level of measurement. Others, like sex, cannot. The decision on levels of measurement is important because it will affect the kinds of statistical analyses that are possible. For example, nominal and ordinal measures – discrete variables – do not normally allow calculations of mean and median, whereas interval and ratio measures – continuous variables – do.

Hofstede's study is a demonstration of the language of operationalization. The language of operationalization involves all the procedures that lead to measurement – from definition of constructs to definition of variables. Hofstede's study has higher-level theoretical statements about relationships and causes – the 'big ideas' statements – such as the relationship between 'cultural values' and 'institutions'. But these big ideas needed to be defined and measured. Hofstede created a large range of variables to study cultural values. He used more than one variable – more than one question in his questionnaire – to measure each dimension. He also collected demographic variables, such as age, sex, education.

Hofstede explicitly addressed the relationship between idiographic and nomothetic approaches to analysing society and attempted to combine both approaches in his own study. His study is 'deductive', with clear ideas about causes and effects and the law-like nature of those causes (to use Holmes's phrase 'all life is a great chain'). The extent to which Hoftstede's general classifications – his quantification – of cultural values are useful or valid is of course open to critique.

MAIN POINTS

- There are three major styles of reasoning in social science research. Deduction involves conclusions about evidence that necessarily occur after reference to certain general laws. Induction involves conclusions about evidence after a build-up of clues. Abduction, which is like guessing, involves conclusions that might still have to be tested with evidence. Each of the styles of reasoning is related to social science research because they are the basis on which we make conclusions about evidence.
- Many of our statements are causal statements but we need to be careful about the logical relationships between cause and effect. In social science there are causal hypotheses and non-causal hypotheses. Correlational hypotheses deal with statements about relationships between variables, but there is no manipulation of variables. Causal hypotheses assume that the independent variable is manipulated and if manipulated will affect the dependent variable.
- Measurement assumes that the phenomenon we want to study is quantifiable – that it has qualities that can be measured at nominal, ordinal, interval or ratio levels. In social science many of the phenomena we try to measure come from everyday life. Nazi Germany's definition of 'Jewishness' and 'Aryan' is an example where the phenomenon itself is socially defined, a part of the everyday life of Germans. The measure of the phenomenon is socially constructed.

REVIEW EXERCISES

1 Find a journal article from a sociology, psychology or media journal that reports on a quantitative research study (this could be the same article you used in last chapter's review exercise). Answer each of these questions:

   (a) What is the hypothesis (if there is one)? Was it causal or non-causal?
   (b) What were the major constructs in the study? How were they defined? Were there problems with the definitions?
   (c) What levels of measurement do you think were used for operationalization of variables?
   (d) What method did the author(s) say they used to collect the data?
   (e) Identify the findings (were there relationships between variables?).

2   Try to put the following hypothesis into operational form:

'The more video games a child watches, the more likely they are to be unsociable'

3   Think of at least two variables and associated levels of measurement for the following constructs:

(a)   boredom
(b)   marital happiness
(c)   deviance
(d)   stress

4   For each of the following measures indicate whether they are a measure on a categorical, ordinal, interval or ratio scale and explain why you have chosen that level of measurement.

(a)   ATM PIN number
(b)   Measuring the length of cars in cms.
(c)   A score on a measure of self-esteem.

REFERENCES

Agresti, A. and Findlay, B. (1997) *Statistical Methods for the Social Sciences*. Prentice Hall: New Jersey.
Babbie, E. (1986) *The Practice of Social Research*. Belmont, CA: Wadsworth.
Chandler, R. (1944) *The Lady in the Lake*. Melbourne: Bolinda Press.
Cliff, N. (1996) *Ordinal Methods for Behavioral Data Analysis*. New Jersey: Lawrence Erlbaum Associates.
Davis, J.A. (1985) *The Logic of Causal Order*. Beverly Hills: Sage.
Doyle, Arthur Conan (1952) *The Complete Sherlock Holmes*. Garden City, New York: Doubleday.
Durkheim, E. (1964) *The Rules of Sociological Method*. New York: Free Press.
Eco, U. (1983) 'Horns, hooves, insteps', in U. Eco and T. Sebeok (eds,) *The Sign of Three: Dupin, Holmes, Pierce*. Bloomington: Indiana University Press.
Friedlander, S. (1997) *Nazi Germany and the Jews*. London: Weidenfeld and Nicolson.
Hacking, I. (1982) 'Language, truth and reason', in M. Hollis and S. Lukes (eds), *Rationality and Relativism*. Oxford: Basil Blackwell.
Hempel, C.G. (1965) *Scientific Explanation: essays in the philosophy of science*. New York: Free Press.
Hofstede, G. (1984) *Culture's Consequences: International differencies in work-related values*. Beverley Hills, CA: Sage.
Higher Education Research & Development (1984) 3(1): 66.
Michell, J. (1997) 'Quantitative science and the definition of measurement in psychology', *British Journal of Psychology*, 88: 355–83.
Michell, J. (1999) *Measurement in Psychology*. Cambridge: Cambridge University Press.

Pierce, C.S. (1955) 'Abduction and induction', in J. Buchler (ed.), *Philosophical Writings of Pierce*, New York: Dover.

Pugh, D. S. and Hickson, D.J. (1989) *Writers on Organizations.* Harmondsworth: Penguin.

Queen, E. (1983) *The Dutch Shoe Mystery.* London: Hamlyn.

Sebeok, T.A. and Umiker-Sebeok, J. (1983) 'You know my method', in U. Eco and T. Sebeok (eds), *The Sign of Three: Dupin, Holmes, Pierce.* Bloomington: Indiana University Press.

Stevens, S.S. (1946) 'On the theory of scales of measurement', *Science*, 103: 667–80.

Stevens, S.S. (1951) 'Mathematics, measurement and psychophysics', in S.S. Stevens (ed), *Handbook of Experimental Psychology.* New York: Wiley. pp. 1–49.

Watson, R., Pattison, P. and Finch, S. (1993) *Beginning Statistics for Psychology.* New York: Prentice Hall.

4

Methods of Inquiry

'It is a capital mistake to theorize before one has data!'

'I have no data yet. It is a capital mistake to theorize
before one has data. Insensibly one begins to twist facts to
suit theories, instead of theories to suit facts'

Sherlock Holmes,
A Scandal in Bohemia

Holmes's methods of detection, he said, were 'an impersonal thing – a thing beyond myself'. The methods of quantitative social science research are similarly a thing apart from us. Our research designs and our research definitions are open to scrutiny and criticism.

Even if we guess in social science research – abduction – we still need to test our guesses, our observations, with data. This is Holmes's point. 'Data' is essential before we start to make 'why' or 'because' conclusions from our observations. But recognizing what is and what is not a clue, data, is itself an art, as we saw in the last chapter. Brother Cadfael, the monk-detective in Ellis Peters' novels, always held back on his decisions on what was and what was not a 'clue'. In *The Sanctuary Sparrow* a young man comes to the abbey seeking sanctuary, safety, after being chased and beaten by men seeking his death. The abbot asks the men why they are chasing the young man: 'My Lord, I will speak for all, I have the right. We mean no disrespect to the abbey or your lordship, but we want that man for murder and robbery done tonight. I accuse him! All here will bear me out. He has struck down my father and plundered his strong-box, and we are come to take him. So if your lordship will allow, we'll rid you of him' (Peters, 1985: 11–12). The abbey looks after the young man while Brother Cadfael investigates. 'We have time, and given time, truth with out', says Cadfael (Peters, 1985: 23). Cadfael senses that the young man is innocent but does not let this influence his thinking on innocence or guilt in his investigation.

Lord Peter Wimsey, Dorothy Sayers' aristocrat detective, is also warned by Parker, his police friend, not to accept uncritically what appears to be obvious. Wimsey is not amused.

'Five-foot ten,' said Lord Peter, 'and not an inch more.' He peered dubiously at the depression in the bed-clothes, and measured it a second time with the gentleman-scout's vademecum. Parker entered this particular in a neat pocket-book.
'I suppose,' he said, 'a six-foot-two man might leave a five-foot-ten depression if he curled himself up.'

Greenfield Medical
ary

lindness / Michelle Alexander.

'Have you any Scotch blood in you, Parker?' inquired his colleague, bitterly.
'Not that I know of,' replied Parker, 'Why?'
'Because of all the cautious, ungenerous, deliberate and cold-blooded devils I know,' said Lord Peter, 'you are the most cautious, ungenerous, deliberate and cold-blooded. Here am I, sweating my brains out to introduce a really sensational incident into your dull and disreputable little police investigation, and you refuse to show a single spark of enthusiasm.'
'Well, it's no good jumping at conclusions.'
'Jump? You don't even crawl distantly within sight of a conclusion. I believe if you caught the cat with her head in the cream-jug, you'd say it was conceivable that the jug was empty when she got there.'
'Well, it would be conceivable, wouldn't it?'
'Curse you,' said Lord Peter. (Sayers, 1989: 54–55)

INVOLVEMENT AND METHOD

A good research design reduces the risk of bias and of 'jumping the gun' on conclusions. A good research design is careful in its decision on what counts as a 'clue'. The men chasing the young man thought that they had the right clues, but they did not. This is not to say that there should be no personal involvement in research. Some methods of detection in social science research involve the researcher as the 'data collecting instrument', such as participant observation. Participant observation – for example living with a traditional society in a remote village in Indonesia – requires a research design. Figure 4.1 provides an overview of the relationship between methods of data collection and involvement. Social surveys and structured interviews involve standardized questions for large groups or populations. Semi-structured interviews and focus groups involve more

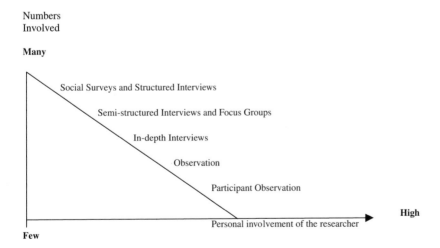

FIGURE 4.1 *Methods of data collection and personal involvement (adapted from Worsley, 1977)*

open questions or prompts. The researcher is not personally involved with participants. In-depth interviews, observation and participant observation, however, assume smaller numbers and may entail greater personal involvement by the researcher.

Notice that 'experiment' has not been included in Figure 4.1. Experiments are a separate case. Small numbers of participants may be involved but the researcher is 'experimenter' rather than 'participant'. A participant observation study, in contrast, involves the researcher directly in the lives of the people that they are studying. The 'data' or 'evidence' in a participant observation may be the accounts of the participants and the accounts of the researcher. These 'accounts' are not necessarily measured. In quantitative studies, such as experiment, the observations are measured.

As we found in Chapter 3, the collection of statistics requires a particular kind of research design. Figure 4.2 is a checklist on this design. We have, to this point, introduced the whole process associated with operationalization, including the literature review. We have not examined, however, the methods themselves or data analysis.

Most modern research methods use a range of data collection techniques – questionnaires, structured interviews, in-depth interviews, observation and content analysis. The three most common forms of data collection are case study, survey and experiment. Case studies investigate 'what is happening' and are very common in policy research and in exploratory

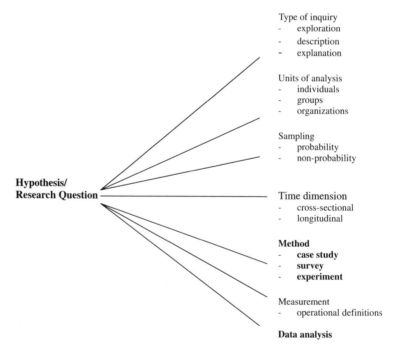

FIGURE 4.2   Checklist for research design

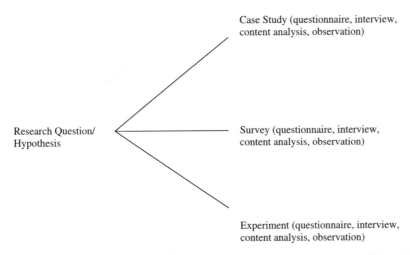

Case Study (questionnaire, interview, content analysis, observation)

Research Question/ Hypothesis

Survey (questionnaire, interview, content analysis, observation)

Experiment (questionnaire, interview, content analysis, observation)

FIGURE 4.3   *Research methods and techniques of data collection (based on DeVaus, 1990: 6. Used by permission)*

work. A survey in comparison can cover a range of issues and normally results in a **variable by case matrix** (person by age, person by education). Questionnaire is one of the most common ways of collecting data for a variable by case data matrix, but it is not the only way. Experiments, like surveys, result in a variable by case matrix. In experiments, however, there is also the intervention by an experimenter. Figure 4.3 provides a summary of the major methods.

In the modern mind experiments are often associated with 'laboratory research', in particular experiments with rats (and white rats at that). But the motivation for 'experiments' has a long history. For Francis Bacon, a philosopher of science, the goal of an experiment is to 'put nature to the test'. Everyone knows that science does experiments, but let us investigate further how experiments differ from other types of methods for analysing observations.

EXPERIMENTAL DESIGN

O, vengeance!
Why, what an ass am I! This is most brave,
That I, the son of a dear father murder'd,
Prompted to my revenge by heaven and hell,
Must, like a whore, unpack my heart with words,
And fall a-cursing like a very drab,
A scullion!
Fie upon't! foh! – About, my brain! I have heard
That guilty creatures, sitting at a play,
Have by the very cunning of the scene
Been struck so to the soul that presently
They have proclaim'd their malefactions;
For murder, though it have no tongue, will speak

With most miraculous organ. I'll have these players
Play something like the murder of my father
Before mine uncle: I'll observe his looks;
I'll test him to the quick: If he but blench,
I know my course. The spirit that I have seen
May be the devil: and the devil hath power
To assume a pleasing shape; yea, and perhaps
Out of my weakness and my melancholy, –
As he is very potent with such spirits, –
Abuses me to damn me: I'll have grounds
More relative than this: – the play's the thing
Wherein I'll catch the conscience of the king.

Hamlet, Act II, Scene II

Hamlet, one of Shakespeare's most famous characters, is not your tradi-tional detective, but he took up the role of detective. Hamlet is not a scien-tist, but he took up the role of experimenter. Hamlet was told by a ghost that the king had killed his father. Hamlet wanted to investigate the claim. Hamlet also wanted to create situations that tested those he thought were participants in the murder. In this case he wanted to create a play for the king which was a recreation of the king's murder of Hamlet's father. The play, Hamlet thought, would get the king to declare his guilt; at least that was the plan.

Hamlet created an experiment – he wanted to manipulate situations in order to observe what the effects would be. He wanted a clear and unam-biguous sign that the king was the murderer. Hamlet found, though, that life is messy. Trying to test everyday life has its downsides.

Columbo, the 1970's television detective, also took an experimental approach to his detection. When he thought that he knew who the murderer was, he would return again and again to the suspect to see what her or his reaction would be. Each time that a suspect thought that Columbo had finished questioning and was about to leave, Columbo would return to ask about '... one more thing'. Columbo's approach was intentionally annoying, leading the suspect to make errors.

Experiments for the scientist are the ideal way of collecting knowledge. They allow for the identification of separate variables and keep all extra-neous – unwanted – variables controlled. An experiment is 'controlled obser-vations of the effects of a manipulated independent variable on some dependent variable' (Schwartz, 1986: 5). We might want to test, for example, a new psychotherapy for people who have a fear of detective fiction. We could find a sample of sufferers, have them undergo the psychotherapy and see if their fear disappears. The problem with this approach is that even if patients improve, we cannot be sure that the therapy was responsible. It may be that people with a fear of detective fiction improve by themselves (spon-taneously) or it may be that something in the therapeutic situation other than psychotherapy itself (having someone care) was responsible for improve-ment. The only way to find out for sure that the psychotherapy was the 'cause' is to control for these extraneous factors by conducting a true experiment. This means creating a second group of people who fear detectives (called the control group) but who do not get the psychotherapy. If they improve as much as the group that does get psychotherapy, then factors other than the psychotherapy may be the answer.

There is always the possibility, of course, that simply getting attention from the therapist affects those with the phobia. This is a 'placebo effect'. A placebo control group, under such circumstances, might also get attention, although not the psychotherapy, from a therapist. If both groups improved under these conditions, then we would probably rule out the psychotherapy as the cause.

Figure 4.4 gives an overview of basic experimental design.

As you can see, the skill of an experiment is in the ability to control variables, including assignment to the experimental and control groups. Ideally, the experimental and control groups need to be the same before the experiment starts. If the phobias of one group are greater than the other, you can see that the results will not be reliable. Participants are often assigned at random to experimental and control groups in the hope that this will result in equal assignment of people to both groups.

The skill of experimental method also includes choosing a study that in fact requires an experimental design. Examine the statements below:

1 Women believe that they are better at dancing than men.
2 Children who are sensitive to poetry in early childhood make better progress in learning to read than those who do not.
3 Remembering a list of items is easier if the list is read four times rather than once.

All these hypotheses involve relationships between variables. However, the last item is most appropriate to experimental method. The first question is about belief, rather than behaviour. The second question involves natural

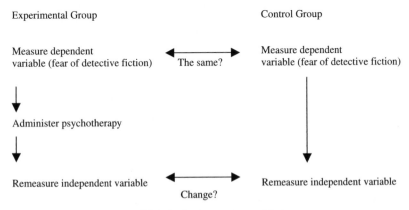

FIGURE 4.4 *Basic experimental design*

language, which, by its nature, is difficult to manipulate. The last question is an obvious candidate for a classical experimental design.

Manipulating and controlling variables in social science research has its limitations. Hamlet was planning to intervene in people's lives to see how they reacted. This raises obvious issues about right and wrong – ethics. You cannot create brain-damaged people, for example, to see how brain damage affects their driving behaviour. In such cases we would be looking at choosing brain-damaged people after they had received the injuries from accident. Such selection is called *ex post facto* experimentation. The nature of the intervention in many ways defines the experimental design that is most appropriate for your study.

There can be little doubt that 'experimental science' has affected research design and society itself and people's assumptions about cause and effect. If experiments can establish causes, then identification of causes can assist all areas of life, including business. But there is a major difference between 'establishing cause' and 'establishing correlation'. Establishing correlation is different from establishing causation. Kaplan (1987: 238–239) demonstrates this in a simple way. He cites a newspaper article on stressfulness of occupations. A study investigated 130 job categories and rated them on stressfulness using Tennessee hospital and death records as evidence of stress-related diseases such as heart attack and mental disorder. Jobs such as unskilled labourer, secretary, assembly-line inspector, clinical lab technician, office manager, foreperson were listed as 'most stressful' and jobs such as clothing sewer, garment checker, stock clerk, skilled craftsperson, housekeeper, farm labourer, were labelled as 'least stressful'. The newspaper advised people to avoid the stressful occupations.

Kaplan (1987) points out that the evidence may not warrant the newspaper's advice. It is possible that diseases are associated with specific occupations, but this does not mean that holding the jobs causes the illnesses. People with a tendency to heart attack, for example, might be more likely to select jobs as unskilled labourers. The direction of causation might be that the state of health causes job selection. Another alternative is that a third variable is having an effect. Income levels, for instance, might affect both stress and illness. 'It is well known that poor people have lower health status than wealthy people' (1987: 239).

Let's look at three possible cases of causation:

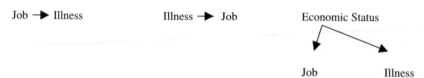

In the first, the job causes the illness. In the second, there is a tendency of people with illnesses to select particular jobs. In the third, economic status, a third variable, affected job choice and illness. To establish causation we would need to know that both X and Y variables co-vary, that X precedes Y in time, and that no other variable is the cause of the change.

At the beginning of the 20th century the idea that experimental social science could easily establish causes was particularly appealing to industries involved in human persuasion. The advertising industry trade journals at the beginning of the century, for example, made it clear that an understanding of the psychology of audiences was essential for advertising success and that this was what their clients were paying for. In 1920, Professor Elton Mayo, chair of Psychology and Ethics at Queensland University, gave the major address at the Second Advertising Men's Conference:

> The ad. expert is an educator in the broadest and highest sense of the term. His task is the persuasion of the people to be civilized. ... You must think for the housewife and if you do that for her and if she finds you are doing it, you will have her confidence. ... It is necessary to understand the fear complexes that are disturbing our social serenity. It is not the slightest use meeting Satanism or Bolshevism by organized rage or hate. Your only chance of dealing with these things is by research, by discovering first and foremost of the cause of this mental condition. (cited in Braverman, 1974: 144–5)

Mayo went on to be internationally famous in the area of industrial psychology and was involved in the famous Hawthorne Experiments in the 1930s and 1940s. The linkage of scientific experimental psychological research to commercial needs was well established in the United States by 1920 with the publication of Walter Dill Scott's *Psychology and Advertising*. In 1922, J.B. Watson, the famous behavioural psychologist, was appointed vice-president of advertising company J. Walter Thompson.

Professor Tasman Lovell was Australia's first chair of psychology in 1923 and joined in the chorus of voices for detailed scientific research of consumer attitudes. An advocate of behavioural psychology, he proclaimed the need for advertising men to 'become versed in the study of instinctive urges, of native tendencies for the need to assert himself, "to keep his end up", which is an aspect of the social instinct that causes him to purchase beyond what is required'. It was not until the mid-1930s, however, when audited circulations of newspapers were available, that advertising firms introduced market analysis on a large scale.

J. Walter Thompson (JWT), an established American advertising agency, employed two psychologists, A.H. Martin and Rudolph Simmat, to oversee advertising research. Martin used mental tests he had developed at Columbia University to measure consumer attitudes towards advertising. In 1927 he established the Australian Institute of Industrial Psychology in Sydney with the support of the University of Sydney's psychology department and the Chamber of Manufacturers. The Institute brought 'local business men in contact with advanced business practices'.

Simmat was appointed research manager for JWT when it established its Australian branch in 1929. JWT standardized art production and research procedures, including segmentation of audiences. The agency divided Australian society into four market **segments**, based on income. Classes A and B were high income housewives. Classes C and D were average or below average income housewives. Class D had 'barely sufficient or even insufficient income to provide itself with the necessities of life. Normally Class D is not greatly important except to the manufacturer of low price, necessary commodities' (Simmat, 1933: 12).

Interviewing techniques were also standardized by Simmat, who had found that experience had shown that women were usually more effective as fieldworkers than men. 'Experiments have indicated that persons with a very high grade of intelligence are unsatisfactory for interviewing housewives ... usually a higher grade of intelligence is required to interview the higher class of housewife than is required to interview the lower grade housewife' (Simmat, 1933: 13).

By 1932 JWT had interviewed 32,000 Australian housewives. Advertising was targeted to specific audiences, with sophistication 'definitely soft-pedaled' for Classes C and D. 'We believe that farce will be more popular with our Rinso [detergent] market than too much subtlety.'

Lever, a soap manufacturer, was one of the first and major supporters of 'scientific advertising'. Simmat expressed Lever's vision when he said that 'Advertising enables the soap manufacturer to regard as his legitimate market every country where people wash or ought to wash'. Lever was the largest advertiser of the period. In 1933–4 Lever bought 183,000 inches of advertising space in metropolitan dailies. Soap, a simple product, crossed all market segments.

The confidence among social scientists at the beginning of the 20th century that they could establish 'cause and effect' was brazen, to say the least. Psychoanalysts also sold their expertise in establishing 'causes' of behaviour. Take, for example, the illustrious Dr Ernest Dichter of the Institute of Motivational Research, who in the 1950s lectured to packed halls of advertisers

and their agents about why people buy their goods. They must have been among the strangest gatherings held for Sydney and Melbourne businessmen. Developing his theme that 'the poorest way to convince is to give facts,' he led his listeners into psycho-analysis, folklore, mythology, and anthropology.

He told them of some of his case histories. There was the Case of the Nylon Bed Sheets. Women would not buy Dupont's nylon non-iron bed sheets, though they were good quality and competitively priced. In despair they consulted Dr. Dichter. He drew up his questionnaire and sent his researchers to interview the women.

After exploring their answers and looking into the sexual and folk associations of bed sheets he discovered that the women were unconsciously jealous of the beautiful blonde lying on the sheets in the advertisements. (Actually, they said their husbands wouldn't like them.) When Grandma was substituted for the blonde, up went the sales. ('I'm surprised,' he said, 'that most of my theories work.') Then there was the Blood and Virility Case. Men had stopped giving blood to the Blood Bank. When consulted, Dr. Dichter discovered they unconsciously feared castration or loss of masculinity. The Bank's name was changed to the Blood Lending Bank, advertisements of beautiful girls trailing masculine blood-donors were prepared, and all went well. (Jones, 1956: 23)

Meanwhile, actual experiments were far more conservative in their conclusions and far more useful than Dichter's theories (guesses?) about the effects of advertising. Carl Hovland's experimental research on the effects of propaganda is a good example. He provided wartime research for the Information and Education division of the US army. Early in 1945 the Army reported that morale was being negatively affected by over-optimism about an early end to the war. The Army issued a directive to the troops informing them of the difficult tasks still ahead. The Army wanted to emphasize that the war could take longer than presumed.

The directive provided an ideal topic for research – which messages are best for influencing people? Hovland et al. (1971) used the directive in an experiment on the effect of presenting 'one side' versus 'both sides' in changing opinions on a controversial subject, namely the time it would take to end the war.

The Armed Forces Radio Services, using official releases, constructed two programmes in the form of a commentator's analysis of the Pacific war. The commentator's conclusion was that it would take at least two years to finish the war in the Pacific after Victory in Europe.

'One Side'. The major topics included in the program which presented only the arguments indicating that the war would be long (hereafter labeled Program A) were: distance problems and other logistical difficulties in the Pacific; the resources and stock piles in the Japanese empire; the size and quality of the main bulk of the Japanese army that we had not yet met in battle; and the determination of the Japanese people. This program ran for about fifteen minutes.

'Both Sides'. The other program (Program B) ran for about nineteen minutes and presented all of these same difficulties in exactly the same way. The additional four minutes in this later program were devoted to considering arguments for the other side of the picture – U.S. advantages and Japanese weaknesses such as: our naval victories and superiority; our previous progress despite a two-front war; our ability to concentrate all our forces on Japan after V-E Day; Japan's shipping losses; Japan's manufacturing inferiority; and the future damage to be expected from our expanding air war. These additional points were woven into the context of the rest of the program, each point being discussed where it was relevant. (1971: 469)

Hovland conducted an initial survey of the troops in the experiment to get an idea of their opinions about the Pacific before hearing the broadcast in order to compare their opinions after the broadcast. The following tables, from Hovland's data, show that the effects were different for the two ways of presenting the messages depending on the initial stand of the listener. Table 4.1 shows that two-sided messages were effective for those who already estimated a short war and one-sided messages were more effective

TABLE 4.1   Effectiveness of Program A and Program B for men with initially unfavourable and men with initially favourable attitudes

	%
Among men whose initial estimate was 'Unfavourable' (estimated a short war)	
Program A (one side only)	36
Program B (both sides)	48
Among men whose initial estimate was 'Favourable' (estimated a long war)	
Program A (one side only)	52
Program B (both sides)	23

TABLE 4.2   Effectiveness of Program A and Program B for men of different educational backgrounds

	%
Among men who did not graduate from high school (changing to a longer estimate)	
Program A (one side only)	46
Program B (both sides)	31
Among men who graduated from high school (changing to a longer estimate)	
Program A (one side only)	35
Program B (both sides)	49

for those who estimated a long war. Table 4.2 shows that two-sided messages are more effective with high school graduates than with nongraduates.

Hovland's research showed that mass-media messages can be used to reinforce and to change attitudes. One-sided messages are most appropriate when people already support a point of view. Two-sided, or balanced, messages are most appropriate when people are better educated and/or opposed to a point of view.

Different Types of Experimental Design

Hovland's study is a classical experiment – an impact study where the participants of the study are directly affected by the independent variables. Estimates of when the war ended were of direct interest to the soldiers concerned.

Not all experiments, however, are of this kind. Many studies involve participants in processes of recognition, recall or evaluation of materials given to them. Such studies have little direct impact on the participants. Impact studies are the ideal, but as Aronson and Merrille Carlsmith (1968: 73–74) point out, 'ethics and good taste confine us to weak empirical operations'.

The basic experimental designs are between-subject (independent) and within-subject (related) design. If two or more totally separate groups of people each receive different levels of the independent variable, then this constitutes a between-subject design. If the same group of people receive all the various levels of the independent variable, then this is an instance of within-subject design. In the television series *The Good Life*, Tom is in the kitchen with three seed boxes. He tells his wife that he is conducting an experiment into the effects of talking to plants. All the boxes contain the same seeds. Box A, says Tom, will be talked to for 10 minutes each morning in a gentle voice. Box B will be shouted at. Box C will not be spoken to. Tom's experiment is a traditional 'between-subject' design (Davis, 1995: 52).

Tom's experiment is a laboratory experiment. Experiments conducted in the natural setting are called field experiments. Bystander apathy, for example, has been an ongoing topic of interest to sociologists. People will often walk past people being robbed or murdered on city streets. Studying such a phenomenon in a laboratory is difficult. Takooshian and Bodinger (1979) organized a national study with volunteers disguised as street roughs. The volunteers staged mock break-ins into cars in busy city streets. In each case, the 'suspect' used a wire coat hanger to force open a car door and then 'stole' TV sets, cameras or other valuable items. The experimenters watched from a hideout not far away. The results for New York showed that in only six out of 214 separate break-ins did passers-by challenge the 'robbers' and then with only very mild queries such as 'Does this car belong to you?' Over 3,000 people walked past the cars. The results from 14 North American cities showed that the intervention rate varied from 0 in Baltimore to 25 per cent in Phoenix, with an average intervention rate of about 10 per cent.

Experiments are attempts to measure observations directly and to ensure that **confounding** and **extraneous** variables are removed. They are direct interventions into people's lives to see how they will react. Direct observations of, and interventions into, large populations are difficult if not impossible in social science research. Survey is one of the most common methods for studying large populations.

SURVEY DESIGN

The time to use surveys is when you cannot observe directly what you want to study. Roman emperors called a census to count the populations under their control because they could not personally observe everyone and wanted to know whom to tax (among other things). These censuses, or surveys, were large but were not designed to answer complex questions about the motivations of the population (for example, 'do you like Emperor Tiberius?').

The *Bills of Mortality* created in Britain in 1594 to survey deaths from plague and other sicknesses are the first modern health statistics. The operational definitions of types of death included: 'Appoplex and suddenly', 'Bedrid', 'Blasted', 'Bloody Flux, Scowring' and 'Flux', 'Drowned', 'Executed', 'Frighted', 'Griping in the Guts', 'Kings Evill', 'Lethargy', 'Spotted Fever and Purples', 'Teeth and Worm', among others. These statistics were, interestingly, concerned not only with recording deaths and baptisms but also with the relationship between the nature of those deaths and God's intentions. Was a drop in baptisms related to punishment by God? Nurses like Florence Nightingale saw the task of quantification as an essentially religious one. She wrote that 'the true foundation of theology is to ascertain the character of God. It is by the aid of statistics that law in the social sphere can be ascertained and codified, and certain aspects of the character of God thereby revealed. The study of statistics is thus a religious service' (cited in David, 1962: 103).

Modern countries conduct regular censuses to count the population. However, when researchers try to elicit complex information through large-scale surveys there is no guarantee that people will provide the information the researcher wants. Karl Marx, the communist writer of the nineteenth century, sent over 20,000 questionnaires to workers to ask them questions about their relationships with their bosses (Marx cited in Bottomore and Rubel, 1956). As far as we know he received no replies.

What is a Survey?

In Chapter 3 we gained an insight into the size and complexity of Geert Hofstede's global survey of employees in a multinational company. A survey is a method of collecting data from people about who they are (education, finances, etc.), how they think (motivations, beliefs, etc.) and what they do (behaviour). Surveys usually take the form of a questionnaire that a person fills out alone or by interview schedule in person or by telephone. The result of the survey is a variable by case data matrix.

There is, of course, massive ongoing collection of data about individuals in modern society – via the internet and other transactions, electronic and otherwise. These data are often used to construct a 'digital persona' – an electronic copy of a person's behaviour and preferences for marketing and other purposes. This is also a form of 'surveying', but, as discussed in Chapter 5, masses of data do not necessarily guarantee meaningful results.

There are three major reasons for conducting surveys in modern societies (Fink and Kosecoff, 1985: 14):

1   Planning a policy or a programme. This can be at a small-scale level where parents might be surveyed about opening hours for a day care centre or employees in a transnational corporation asked how they feel about their boss.
2   Evaluating the effectiveness of programmes to change people's knowledge, attitudes, health, or welfare. This could include, for example, major media campaigns, such as quit smoking. Such campaigns, which can cost millions of dollars, require evaluation of their effectiveness.
3   Assisting research and planning generally. This can include everything from a sociologist's concern with measuring social inequality to the census.

Designing questions in a questionnaire requires skill in understanding levels of measurement (and the statistical purposes for which the questions are going to be put); using simple language (and pre-testing that language); and administration.

The Variable in Question

The questions in your questionnaire are your variables. Your operational definitions – your choices on how to measure your constructs – should be reflected in the variables in your questionnaire. If you have the hypothesis 'men are more likely than women to watch television', then these two variables will be present in the questionnaire. A survey, of course, might be based on a research question – a general statement about an area of interest, rather than a specific hypothesis(es). In either case you will be dealing with variables.

The questions in a questionnaire will reflect the appropriate levels of measurement necessary for further statistical analysis. These levels of measurement – nominal, ordinal, interval and ratio – were discussed in Chapter 3. The levels of measurement also reflect the nature of the phenomenon you are studying. There are limits on what numbers can do with phenomena.

Nominal Variables/Questions

Nominal-level questions are those designed to elicit responses that take categorical form. For example, if you respond 'male' to the question 'Are you male or female?', then you have provided a response to a nominal rating scale. There is no meaningful 'distance' between the numbers '1' to represent 'male' and '2' to represent 'female', except that the categories are different. It is possible to add up each of the categories and get frequencies, but there is no such thing as 'average gender' and you cannot subtract one male from one female or multiply or divide one male and one female. Notice also that you can never say there is nothing of the phenomenon. You are always either male or female. The questions below are examples of nominal-level measurements.

What type of dwelling is this residence?
1 Separate house, semi-detached,
   row/terrace, townhouse, etc.
      One storey   (   )
      Two or more storeys   (   )
2 Unit/Flat
      In a one or two storey block   (   )
      In a three or more storey block   (   )
3 Other (Please specify)..

Is any adult currently studying?
Yes   (   )
No   (   )

Note that question 3 is **open-ended** while the other questions are **closed-ended**. Closed-ended questions provide only fixed choices for the respondents. However, question 3 can be **post-coded** because each of the answers could be classified and coded as nominal data.

Ordinal Variables/Questions

Ordinal-level questions require people to answer in rank order. Ordinal questions have a 'more or less' aspect to them. Many social science constructs are measured at the ordinal or rank level. A 'rank' does not tell you how far apart intervals are. For example, if you hear that the horse race ends with first, second and third, you have a rank but you do not know the distance between the horses. The question below is an example of ranking.

Please rank the following four items according their importance to you in your use of the telephone. The top ranked should be assigned the number 1 and the lowest rank the number 4.
Business calls   (   )
Talking to friends   (   )
Talking to relatives   (   )
Information services   (   )

Interval Variables/Questions

Intelligence Quotient (IQ) is often given as an example of an interval-level measure. There is always something of the phenomenon and the distances between the intervals are supposed to be known. With interval level the numbers attached to a variable imply not only that, for example, 3 is more than 2 and 2 is more than 1 but also that the size of the interval between 3 and 2 is the same as the interval between 2 and 1. A question that asked people whether they strongly agreed, disagreed, strongly disagreed is often treated as an interval-level measurement in modern research even though it looks 'ordinal'. This is where it can get tricky because the issue for the researcher is whether the distance between the interval – the distance between 'agree' and 'disagree', for example – is meaningful. One person's 'agree' might be another person's 'disagree'.

The question below, 'what is your household's annual income?', would be described by Fink and Cosecoff (1985) as an interval-level question. Using such data to make conclusions about other constructs, however, needs care. If, for example, we tried to measure social status using income, then 'ranges' can be deceptive. A person with a salary of $20,000 would be in a very different 'status' compared with a person on '$50,000', but the $30,000 difference means less as we go up the scale. A person on $130,000, for instance, is unlikely to be in a significantly different status group compared with a person on $150,000.

What is your household's annual income?

Less than $3,000	( )	$50,001–$60,000	( )
$3,001–$5,000	( )	$60,001–$70,000	( )
$5,001–$8,000	( )	$70,001–$80,000	( )
$8,001–$12,000	( )	$80,001–$90,000	( )
$12,001–$16,000	( )	$90,001–$100,000	( )
$16,001–$20,000	( )	$100,001–$120,000	( )
$20,001–$25,000	( )	More than $120,000	( )
$25,001–$30,000	( )	Prefer not to say	( )
$30,001–$35,000	( )	Not applicable	( )
$35,001–$40,000	( )		
$40,001–$50,000	( )		

Ratio Variables/Questions

Ratio-level measures, as discussed in the previous chapter, have a true zero point. The question below is a ratio-level question. With this ratio-level question it is possible to say which households have twice the number of radios compared with other households, something that you cannot do with lower levels of measurement.

How many radios are there in this dwelling? (............)

Understanding levels of measurement is partly an understanding of the phenomenon you are studying. Sex, as a variable, for example, cannot be operationalized as a ratio-level question. A 'zero' is meaningless in this context. Income, however, can be operationalized at all levels of measurement. You can ask the question 'Do you have an income?' with the reply 'Yes' or 'No'. You have operationalized income at the nominal level. You lose a lot of information, though, in such a question.

Multiple-Item Scales

Multiple-item scales have been developed to provide a more sophisticated way of measuring people's underlying attitudes. There are three major types of scale – differential scales, cumulative scales and summative scales. Each scale entails different assumptions about the relationship between the responses an individual provides and the measurement of the underlying attitude.

Differential Scales

Thurstone (1929) created differential scales. People are assumed to agree with only those items whose position is close to their own. Statements related to the attitude are gathered and submitted to 'judges' who classify

TABLE 4.3   Examples from Thurstone's differential scale

Scale value	Item
1.2	I believe the church is a powerful agency for promoting both individual and social righteousness
3.3	I enjoy my church because there is a spirit of friendliness there
4.5	I believe in what the church teaches but with mental reservations
9.2	I think the church seeks to impose a lot of worn-out dogmas and medieval superstitions
11.0	I think the church is a parasite on society

TABLE 4.4   Examples from Bogardus Social Distance scale

	To close kinship by marriage	To my club as personal chum	To my street as neighbour	To employment in my occupation	To citizenship in my country	As visitors only to my country	Would exclude from my country
English	1	2	3	4	5	6	7
Black	1	2	3	4	5	6	7
French	1	2	3	4	5	6	7
Chinese	1	2	3	4	5	6	7
Russian	1	2	3	4	5	6	7

the items according to their position on a dimension. Table 4.3 shows Thurstone's study of attitudes towards the Church. Items on which judges fail to agree are rejected. Items representing a wide range of scale values form the scale and are then presented to respondents. Thurstone's items have a definite position on the scale.

Cumulative Scales
Cumulative scales allow agreement and disagreement for each item. The Bogardus Social Distance scale (Bogardus, 1925) was one of the earliest scales of this type. Table 4.4 shows how the cumulative scale works. A person who circles number 3 in respect to some group, indicating willingness to have them in the street as a neighbour, would also be willing, one would think, to allow them as citizens of the country. The scale score is defined as the total number of items agreed with.

Summative Scales
Summative scales allow agreement and disagreement on individual items. Respondents normally respond to an item with: (1) strongly disagree; (2) disagree; (3) agree; (4) strongly agree. The scale score is obtained by summing the responses to each item (taking into account sign reversal for negative items). Likert (1932) scales are the most common form of summative scale.

Table 4.5 is taken from the Mach IV scale of Christie and Geis (1970). Mach IV is a measure of Machiavellianism and the desire to manipulate others. The positive items (+), which might run Strongly Agree (4),

TABLE 4.5   *Selected examples from Christie and Geis's Likert scale*

Item	Strongly Agree	Agree	Disagree	Strongly Disagree
The best way to handle people is to tell them what they want (+)				
It is wise to flatter important people (+)				
When you ask someone to do something for you, it is best to give the real reasons for wanting it rather than the reasons which might carry more weight (−)				

Agree (3), Disagree (2), Strongly Disagree (1), are balance by negative items reversing the scores, Strongly Agree (1), Agree (2), Disagree (3), Strongly (4). Each of the items relates to the construct of interest – manipulation. Only three of the Mach IV items are presented in Table 4.5.

Item scales are subject to special kinds of bias or error. Halo bias refers to the tendency for overall positive or negative evaluations of the person (or thing) being rated. Generosity error refers to raters' overestimation of desirable qualities of people that the rater likes. Contrast error refers to how some raters seem to avoid extreme response categories (such as strongly disagree). There are tests that have been created to check the validity and reliability of items in scales and these should be used in the pilot phase.

The Words in the Question

Inspector Clouseau, the comic-clumsy French detective played by Peter Sellers, often gets into trouble with pronunciation. He pronounces 'monkeys' 'minkeys', 'phones' 'ferns' and 'room' 'rhum'. People do not understand what he is saying, until he clarifies what he has said. Questionnaires have the same problem. You think that the sentence you have written will be understood, but it isn't.

The same question worded in two different ways can produce different results. Howard Schuman and Stanley Presser of the Survey Research Center at the University of Michigan replicated in 1974 a 1940 experiment with the following outcomes:

'Do you think the United States should forbid public speeches against democracy?' Forbid: 28% Not forbid: 72%
'Do you think the United States should allow public speeches against democracy?' Not allow: 44% Allow: 56% (Schuman and Presser, 1977)

The words we use in a sentence can have a dramatic effect on the result. In this case, the word 'forbid' raised concerns among a large proportion of the respondents to the survey. People may also not understand the meanings of the words. Cannell and Kahn (1968) cited 1960s estimates that the average American knew fewer than 10 per cent of the words in the English language. Wording for questions in a questionnaire is not only a matter of coming up with good questions that relate to the research question or hypothesis of interest but coming up with good questions that can be understood. An important part of questionnaire design includes understanding of the **frame of reference** of the people you are studying. Frame of reference – everyday life – involves understanding the ambiguity of language and the fact that each individual necessarily interprets spoken or written communication from his or her own experience and personal viewpoint.

There are three ways of dealing with frame of reference: ignore it, ascertain it, or control it.

Bancroft and Welch (1946: 540–549) provide a classic illustration of the effect of frame of reference on responses to questionnaires. They found that the series of questions used by the Bureau of Census in the US to ascertain the number of people in the labour market consistently underestimated the number of employed persons. When asked the question: 'Did you do any work for pay or profit last week?' respondents reported in terms of what they considered their major activity, in spite of the explicit defining phrase 'for pay or profit'. Young people going to school considered themselves to be students even if they were also employed on a part-time basis. Women who cooked, cleaned house, and raised children spoke of themselves as housewives, even if they also did some work for pay outside the home. The answer to this problem was to ascertain the frame of reference and to control it. People were asked first what their major activity was; those who gave nonworker responses were asked whether, in addition to their major activity, they did any work for pay. This provided a simple but effective solution.

Once the frame of reference is understood it is important to write questions that avoid any additional bias. DeVaus (1985: 83) provides a simple checklist for the wording of questions:

1 Is the language simple? Do not use jargon or technical terms that people will not understand. A question such as 'Is your household a patriarchy?' will be understood by some people and not others.
2 Can the question be shortened?
3 Is the question double-barrelled? Double-barrelled questions are those which ask more than one question in the same sentence. 'How often do you visit your parents?' should be broken into a question about the mother and a question about the father.
4 Is the question leading? Questions that make people feel that they have to answer in a particular way are 'leading'. 'Do you support the defence of our country?' is loaded. A person would feel obliged to say 'yes'. A question starting 'Do you agree that . . . ' also gives respondents a feeling that they are giving a wrong answer if they say 'no'.
5 Is the question negative? Using 'not' in a sentence can be misleading. The question 'Marijuana should not be decriminalized' – agree/dis-

agree should be written 'Marijuana use should remain illegal' – agree/disagree.

6 Does the respondent have the necessary knowledge? A question that asks 'Do you agree with the government's handling of the waterfront crisis?' requires knowledge about the crisis. A 'filter' question is used to check whether respondents have the knowledge. 'Do you know about the current waterfront crisis?'

7 Will the words have the same meaning for everyone? If words have different meanings for different subcultural groups, then avoid them.

8 Is there prestige bias in the question? People sometimes distort answers to impress the interviewer. They might exaggerate income, education or minimize their age. There is no simple solution to this. It is called a social desirability response set. These 'sets' can sometimes be identified in analysis. However, avoiding leading questions will reduce this type of bias.

9 Is the question ambiguous? The longer the sentence and the more complex the wording in a question, the greater the possibility of bias.

10 Direct and indirect questions. Some topics are extremely sensitive and, in fact, may not be allowed by an ethics committee. 'Have you had an affair that your partner does not know about?' is not only direct, it is biased in other ways (e.g. the possibility of prestige bias). If a question cannot be asked directly, then indirect questions need to be created.

11 Is the frame of reference for the question clear? The question 'what is your occupation?', as an open-ended question, is reasonable, but may receive the reply 'engineer'. There are many types of engineer. Providing categories of occupation (e.g. as defined by the census) would assist here. Asking the question 'How often do you visit your father?' is also reasonable, but more specific information on frequency is required.

12 Does the question artificially create opinions? You should, where appropriate, give people the option of 'don't know' or 'prefer not to say'.

13 Is personal or impersonal wording preferable? You can ask people how they feel about something, or how they think other people feel about something. The choice of 'personal' or 'impersonal' approaches to wording will depend on the researcher's interests.

14 Is the question wording unnecessarily detailed or objectionable? Questions about precise age, for example, might cause problems. This is often solved by putting age into ranges.

Basic demographic questions have often been tested and re-tested by major government census and statistics agencies in their own survey work. These agencies publish guides to questionnaire design and the operational definitions used in their own questions.

Administering the Questionnaire

Administration of the questionnaire involves layout, decisions on length of questionnaire, types of questions to be asked, implementing the survey, monitoring the quality of answers, response rates and ethics issues. Poor administration of a questionnaire can lead to low response rates, poor quality responses and poor data generally. The questionnaire is also an 'ambassador' for the research project. If respondents feel that you have not taken care in its design, then it is unlikely that they will be motivated to fill it out.

Layout

The layout of a questionnaire includes:

1 General introduction (the purpose of the questionnaire, how people were selected, assurance of confidentiality and how and where to return a mailed questionnaire).
2 Question instructions (how questions are to be answered).
3 Order (simple questions should go first, complex questions last; concrete questions first, abstract questions last).
4 Creating a numerical code (a scale or other system of numbers into which the recorded responses are to be translated).

A general introduction tells respondents about the study, but it might also be supplemented by a letter requiring signed informed consent. In most cases, return of a questionnaire counts as 'informed consent'. However, many studies seek signed informed consent. Appendix I is an example of a proforma letter for informed consent, produced by Murdoch University ethics committee. Informed consent can include agreement to publication of data.

Well-formatted questions assist response rate and accuracy of answers. There is a variety of answer formats. Whichever format you choose you should be (a) consistent in use of that format and (b) consistent in the type of response required for that format (for example, don't combine ticking, circling, crossing out within the same format). Figure 4.5 is an example of some commonly used formats. Contingency questions are an often-used format. Figure 4.6 is an example of a contingency question. Contingency questions have obvious benefits in reducing confusion.

Contingency and 'go to' questions enable efficient use of space.

[ ] Agree	☐ Agree	( ) Agree
[ ] Disagree	☐ Disagree	( ) Disagree
[ ] Undecided	☐ Undecided	( ) Undecided

FIGURE 4.5   *Different answering formats*

Were you born in Britain?

1.   ( ) Yes (go to Q2)

   ( ) No

(a) Where were you born?_____

(b) How many years have you lived here?_____

Go to Question 2

FIGURE 4.6   *Contingency questions*

Well-formatted questions improve the probability of getting accurate responses. A coding book for a questionnaire involves assigning numbers to the responses for efficient recording of appropriate and inappropriate responses and non-responses. After people have answered questions, the researcher needs a system for transferring those data from the questionnaire itself to the computer. This is the role of a coding column.

Table 4.6 provides a sample coding column. The first numbers in the 'official use only' column, will identify the questionnaire (not the respondent). The other numbers in the column identify the responses to each question.

You will need to decide on a coding system for each question. This coding system will assist entry of the data into the computer. Your 'code' for the first question, for example, has five possibilities. Your code of 1 to 5 would cover an answer in any of the five options to question 1. There are other possible outcomes, however, including non-responses and inappropriate responses. A code for non-response may be 9 and a code for an inappropriate response may be 0. '1' in your computer would represent the response to 'one storey separate house, semi-detached, row/terrace, townhouse, etc.', '2', 'two or more storey separate house, semi-detached, row/terrace, townhouse, etc.', and so on.

Length of Questionnaire

There are no set rules for the length of a mailed self-administered questionnaire or the length of an interview. Dillman (1978) found that the optimal length for questionnaires to the general public was about 12 pages or 125 items. Response rates drop rapidly if a questionnaire is longer. Surveys for special groups, however, may be longer. A survey of social workers about their profession, for example, is of special interest to the survey workers. Babbie (1986: 22) says that a 50 per cent response rate for a questionnaire is adequate, 60 per cent is good and 70 per cent very good. Response

TABLE 4.6   *Sample questionnaire and coding column*

			For official use only Ident.____ 1–3
Q1 What type of dwelling is this residence?			_4
1 Separate house, semi–detached, row/terrace, townhouse, etc.			
One storey	(	)	
Two or more storeys	(	)	
2 Unit/Flat			
In a one or two storey block	(	)	
In a three or more storey block	(	)	
3 Other (Please specify)...........................	(	)	
Q2 Is any adult currently studying?			
Yes	(	)	_5
No	(	)	

Q3   What is your household's annual income?

					_6
Less than $3,000	( )	$50,001 – $60,000	( )		
$3,001 – $5,000	( )	$60,001 – $70,000	( )		
$5,001 – $8,000	( )	$70,001 – $80,000	( )		
$8,001 – $12,000	( )	$80,001 – $90,000	( )		
$12,001 – $16,000	( )	$90,001 – $100,000	( )		
$16,001 – $20,000	( )	$100,001 – $120,000	( )		
$20,001 – $25,000	( )	More than $120,000	( )		
$25,001 – $30,000	( )	Prefer not to say	( )		
$30,001 – $35,000	( )	Not applicable	( )		
$35,001 – $40,000	( )				
$40,001 – $50,000	( )				

Q4 How many radios are there in this dwelling?	(.....)	__7–8

rates for mailed questionnaires increase, however, if there is a follow-up with respondents who have not returned their questionnaire. Response rates for telephone and face-to-face interviews tend to be higher than mailed questionnaires. More complex questions are also possible in face-to-face and telephone interviews.

Interview as Measurement

Telephone and face-to-face interviews allow greater flexibility in presenting information to respondents. The research design for interview schedules is similar to mailed questionnaires but includes additional issues of complexity of questions, response biases in interview situations, and monitoring interviewer progress. The general procedures for structured interviews involves:

1   Creating or selecting an interview schedule (set of questions, statements, pictures) and a set of rules or procedures for using the schedule
2   Conducting the interview

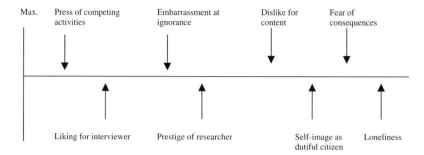

FIGURE 4.7 *Factors affecting people's motivation to provide complete and accurate information to the interviewer (adapted from Cannell and Kahn, 1968: 539)*

3 Recording the responses
4 Creating a numerical code (a scale or other system of numbers into which the recorded responses are to be translated)
5 Coding the interview responses.

The general goals of interviewing are to create a positive atmosphere, ask the questions properly, obtain an adequate response, record the response and avoid biases. Interviewer bias includes attitudes, interviewer characteristics (e.g. age, sex, ethnic background) and interviewer perceptions of the situation.

Figure 4.7 shows the competing forces at play in the interview situation. From the interviewee's perspective, press of competing activities, embarrassment at ignorance, dislike for content, and fear of consequences in answering in the wrong way are at a maximum in an interview situation. The research design should maximize the forces that are at a minimum. Understanding frame of reference and good design are, of course, factors that maximize those forces.

A **pilot study** – a preliminary test of a questionnaire or interview schedule – helps to identify problems and benefits associated with the design. It also helps the researcher to get a better understanding of the frame of reference relevant to the questionnaire and question wording. Figure 4.8 provides a checklist for questionnaire design.

Good design, measurement and administration of a questionnaire or an interview schedule reduce bias and possible errors. These are the keys to enhanced construct and internal validity.

VALIDITY

A 'method' is not a neutral framework – it embodies the procedures you use to collect and analyse evidence. We could apply the method and get bad results. We could apply it again and get the same bad results. Our methods

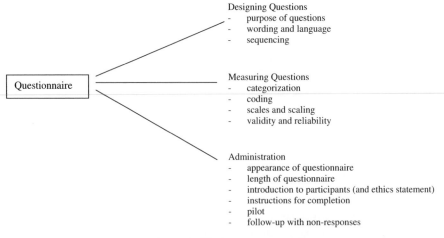

Questionnaire

Designing Questions
- purpose of questions
- wording and language
- sequencing

Measuring Questions
- categorization
- coding
- scales and scaling
- validity and reliability

Administration
- appearance of questionnaire
- length of questionnaire
- introduction to participants (and ethics statement)
- instructions for completion
- pilot
- follow-up with non-responses

FIGURE 4.8   *Checklist for questionnaire design*

might be reliable, therefore, but not valid. Issues of validity are a part of research design.

Detectives have an interest in whether clues are real clues and whether clues really do solve the problem they are studying. Do the clues represent what you think that they represent? William of Baskerville, the monk-detective in Umberto Eco's book, *The Name of the Rose*, was expert at identifying clues but, as this discussion with Adso, his subordinate novice, shows, he was not so confident about his judgements about the overall meaning of the clues.

'But master,' I ventured, sorrowfully, 'you speak like this now because you are wounded in the depths of your spirit. There is one truth, however, that you discovered tonight, the one you reached by interpreting the clues you read over the past few days. Jorge has won, but you have defeated Jorge because you exposed his plot ... '

'There was no plot,' William said, 'and I discovered it by mistake.'

The assertion was self-contradictory, and I couldn't decide whether William really wanted it to be. 'But it was true that the tracks in the snow led to Brunellas,' I said, 'it was true that Adelmo committed suicide, it was true that Venantius did not drown in the jar, it was true that the labyrinth was laid out in the way you imagined it, it was true that one entered the finis Africae by touching the word "quatuor," it was true that the mysterious book was by Aristotle ... I could go on listing all the true things you discovered with the help of your learning ... '

'I have never doubted the truth of signs, Adso; they are the only things man has with which to orient himself in the world. What I did not understand was the relation among signs. I arrived at Jorge through an apocalyptic pattern that seemed to underlie all the crimes, and yet it was accidental. I arrived at Jorge seeking one criminal for all the crimes and we discovered that each crime was committed by a different person, or by no one. I arrived at Jorge pursuing the plan of a perverse and rational mind, and there was no plan ...' (Eco, 1980: 491–492).

In social science research, just as in detective fiction, what you think you have got right at one level may be wrong at another level. You might find a specific clue and understand its local significance but get the big picture wrong. We want our conclusions to be valid and reliable. Validity in quantitative research is the extent to which your measures do, in fact, measure the constructs of interest to the research. If I tell you that I have measured 'sex' by 'black' and 'white', then you would quite rightly tell me that you have problems with the validity of my definitions. You will tell me that black and white do not measure sex.

There are three major kinds of validity: construct validity, internal validity and external validity. Construct validity is the extent to which your constructs are successfully operationalized and represent the phenomenon you want to study. Internal validity is the extent to which your research design really allows you to draw conclusions about the relationship between variables. External validity is the extent to which your sample is genuinely representative of the population from which you have drawn it. Table 4.7, adapted from Judd et al. (1991: 55), provides a good example of what happens when a test is not measuring what it is supposed to measure. For example, in Operational Definition 1 we have given an English (untranslated) IQ test to French students. In Operational Definition 2 we have provided a translation. In Operational Definition 3 we have provided the test through interviews. Jacques, as you can see, did well under the English IQ test. The reason? He was probably good at English. There is, however, consistency between the second and third measures. The main sources of bias and error in the measurements are knowledge of English in measure 1 and conversational skills for measure 2. Robert, for example, did better in the French translation of the IQ test compared with his interview. It is likely that it was the interview that affected his ability to do the IQ test.

Maximizing construct validity and internal validity – ensuring that our measures do, indeed, measure what we say they do – reduces the error and

TABLE 4.7   Rank order of French high school students' intelligence scores obtained with three hypothetical measures

Operational Definition 1 English IQ test	Operational Definition 2 French translation	Operational Definition 3 French interviews
Jacques	Pierre	Pierre
Carole	Marie	Marie
Marie	Jeanne	Jeanne
Marianne	Jacques	Jacques
Lisa	Lisa	Lisa
Pierre	Carole	Carole
Jeanne	Robert	Marianne
Robert	Marianne	Robert

(Used by permission)

the bias that might affect our conclusions. Research studies can use poor operational definitions and still be reliable – give us consistent results – but not be valid. We want reliability in our study, but reliability should not come at the cost of validity.

Experiments in particular seek to maximize internal validity. However, experiments are also susceptible to their own problems of internal validity. There may be testing or 'instrument' effects, where the test materials themselves might affect what people do. There are also maturation effects, where time may affect the nature of the experiment. Let's look at 'order effects' and 'carry over' effects as an example (Davis, 1995: 63–64). Tasks in an experiment which are completed serially, one after another, can create 'order effects'. A person is quite likely to gain experience with the nature of the task. If the performance of one task carries over to another task in an experiment, then there may also be 'carry over' effects.

Davis (1995: 64) uses a Piagetian experiment to demonstrate the difference between order and carry-over effects. In one Piagetian experiment, children under the age of five often report that the number of objects in a row actually increases simply because an adult (acting as experimenter) spreads the row of objects out so that the row appears longer. If the experimenter next uses a teddy bear to spread the row of objects, however, the children do not say that the number of objects has increased. If the teddy bear is used first in the experiment to spread the objects, then the children are more likely to give correct responses: 'it is not that children show an improvement from first to second task but that they show improvement only with a particular sequence of conditions' (1995: 64). The carry-over effects in this case are of interest because they affect the experiment. However, they are also of theoretical interest.

Internal validity addresses problems in operational definition and the relationships between variables. Problems associated with sampling, however, raise a different set of problems. External validity is associated with sampling. Procedures for sampling enhance external validity.

EXTERNAL VALIDITY AND SAMPLING

Sampling in social science research is a technique, a procedure, for selecting a subset of units of analysis from a population. Good sampling achieves representativeness. Detectives in detective fiction are always trying to judge representativeness – for example, whether the crook they are looking for belongs to a typical class of crook or that a particular character is representative of a particular kind of behaviour. In Chandler's *Lady of the Lake*, Marlowe is quick to offer his judgements about whether particular kinds of behaviour are stereotypical, even when those judgements have an undertone of sexism: 'I get a very vague idea of Mrs. Kingsley – that she is young, pretty, reckless, and wild. That she drinks and does dangerous things when she drinks. That she is a sucker for the men and might take up with a stranger who might turn out to be a crook. Does that fit?' He [Mr. Kingsley] nodded. 'Every word of it' (Chandler, 1944: 23).

Working out whether a sample is the right sample is not a simple matter in quantitative research. You need to decide what your population is and whether each element of that population can be identified and listed.

Population and Sampling Frame

Constructs are defined and measured by the social scientist. Samples, similarly, are defined and measured by the social scientist. The social scientist uses statistics to make judgements, inferences, about the phenomenon that he or she is studying. The social scientist uses samples and sample statistics to make inferences about the populations from which they are drawn.

Populations are operationally defined by the researcher. They must be accessible and quantifiable and related to the purpose of the research. 'All households in London' is a definition of a population, with households as the unit of analysis. But what is a 'household'? Is it any dwelling, including the boat in the backyard that your brother lives in? Is it Buckingham Palace? If all of these examples are 'households', then these need to be included in the definition of the population. If a sample of households was drawn from London, then 'London' needs to be defined. Is London defined by local council boundaries? Is it defined by census boundaries?

When you have decided on all these definitions, then every household in London that you have defined as a household belongs on your list. That list is called a *sampling frame*.

Simple Random Sampling

You can number each household, if you wish, and put them in a hat (a big hat in this case). Let us say that you drew out 10 households (a sample). You know that there was no bias in your choice. Each element, each household, in your sampling frame had an equal chance of being chosen. This is called a **probability or random sample**. You could also use a table of random numbers. For example, a researcher who wants to analyse 15 households out of 100 households would number each household from 00 to 99. The researcher would then select 15 numbers from a table of random numbers, such as the truncated listing in Table 4.8. You can start anywhere in the table of random numbers and then proceeding up, down or diagonally, select the 15 numbers needed. In this case, the selection starting from 28 downwards would be 28, 36, 77, 17, and so on.

By chance, however, we might find that all 15 households you pulled from the hat are boats. We have not represented all households, only boats. In the study we may require, therefore, stratified random sampling. We break up the sampling frame into different strata and then conduct a simple random sample.

TABLE 4.8   *Table of random numbers*

2	8	4	9	8	8	9	9	5	5
3	6	1	9	0	3	0	1	1	1
7	7	9	9	7	8	3	3	3	2
1	7	6	9	2	4	1	8	6	7

Stratified Random Sampling

We could split up households in the list by type of household into single-level households, double-level household, boats, and other classifications. There may be very few boats-as-households in the population – 10 per cent. If we wanted to represent that 10 per cent in our sampling, then 10 per cent of our sample would be boats. This is a proportionate stratified random sample, where we represent each type of household proportionately. A simple random sample from each separate list of types of household would be required. Sometimes we might want to over-represent a particular stratum, especially if there are very low numbers. For example, you might decide that people living on boats are of special interest. This is **disproportionate stratified random sampling.**

Multi-Stage Cluster Sampling

Large-scale, national studies often use a form of cluster sampling called multi-stage cluster sampling. Normally we select one unit at a time in probability sampling. This requires a complete list of the units of analysis. Sometimes there is no way to create a list. In these cases we use a procedure known as cluster sampling. In cluster sampling we select groups or categories. For example, following Figure 4.9, we can break London up into suburbs and randomly sample those suburbs. We could then break up those suburbs into census collectors' districts (about 400 households) and then randomly select those districts. We could then select streets and **systematically** sample those streets. A systematic sample is when every *n*th unit of analysis is selected – every second house in the street, for instance. Once we have selected our sample of households, we would then select our demographic quota from those households (people of a certain age or sex, etc.). In order to randomly select our participants we could again use a table of random numbers designed for this purpose (Table 4.9). For example, the interviewer could ask 'How many people are there in your home aged 15 or older?' If the first participant says 'three people', then according to Table 4.9 the second oldest person is chosen.

Simple, stratified and multi-stage cluster sampling are all forms of probability sampling. Going to a shopping mall and talking to a person whom you think would be useful for your study is NOT random sampling – that person did not have an equal and known chance of being selected.

Why do we need probability sampling? Good sampling reduces the chance that we have picked the wrong people or unit of analysis for our

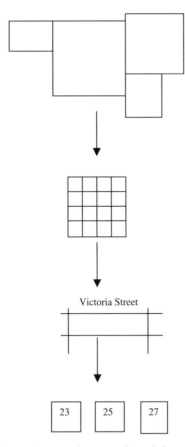

FIGURE 4.9   *Multi-stage cluster sampling – following the census tracts*

study. Good sampling reduces error and maximizes external validity. The statistics we use for analysis of samples also require probability sampling. Statistics that make judgements about the relationship between samples and their population are called **inferential statistics**. We will talk about inferential statistics in Chapter 6.

Table 4.10 provides a summary of the probability sampling procedures. Simple random sampling is good where there is a high degree of homogeneity in the defined population. Stratified random sampling is good where there is a high degree of heterogeneity. Cluster sampling is an economical way to get access to populations, but increases error because we are dealing with groups.

Sample Size

A large sample is no guarantee of accuracy. The *Literary Digest* in the United States regularly polled its readers between 1916 and 1932 and it

TABLE 4.9   *Random selection of households for interview*

	No. of people in household				
	1	2	3	4	5
Person to interview	1	2	2	4	3
		1	1	2	5
			3	1	4
				3	1
					2

TABLE 4.10   *Summary of sampling procedures*

Design	Description	Benefit
Simple random	All units of analysis are known and each have an equal chance of selection	Generalizability of findings
Stratified random	Population is divided into strata and units then selected:	Most efficient of the designs
Proportionate	In proportion to the original strata	Sampling frame for each stratum required
Disproportionate	Based on criteria where different proportions may be required	Good for representing strata that have small numbers
Cluster sampling	Based on groups or geographical clusters with all members in each cluster randomly selected	Costs of data collection reduced, but increased chance of error

regularly picked the winners of presidential elections. The magazine mailed out ballots to over 10 million residential telephone users and, in later years, car owners. The size of the sample was thought to explain its success and was often called 'uncanny', 'amazingly accurate', and 'infallible' (Hunt, 1985: 122). In 1936, however, the *Literary Digest's* reputation suffered a blow: 2,376,523 ballots said that Franklin Roosevelt would get only 41 per cent of the vote. In fact Roosevelt got 61 per cent of the vote.

The sample, in this case, was drawn from an unrepresentative group – those who had telephones and cars. The Gallup and Fortune surveys came close to the final result because they tried to sample proper proportions of people at every social and geographic level.

In simple experimental research with strict controls, successful research may be conducted with samples as small as 10 to 20 in size. In most experimental research the use of samples of 30 or larger is recommended. In multivariate research the sample size should be several times (more than 10 times) as large as the number of variables. There are few occasions in behavioural research where samples smaller than 30 or larger than 500 in size can be justified. The more complex your study, of course, and the more complex your requirements, the more expensive your sampling is going to be.

Non-Probability Sampling

Not all populations defined by a researcher are easily accessible or easily quantifiable. For example, 'all heroin users in the United Kingdom' is an operational definition for a particular kind of population, but it is unlikely that you could find them all or list them all (a sampling frame). You could, of course, define your population as 'all convicted heroin users in British prisons', in which case the establishment of a sampling frame becomes more feasible (assuming ethics approval).

Researchers who cannot ensure that every unit in their population has an equal chance of being selected, or who simply don't need a sampling frame, often use non-probability techniques. The major non-probability techniques are judgement, opportunistic and snowball sampling. *Judgement sampling* involves the selection of the units of analysis according to criteria established by the researcher (e.g. age, sex, occupation). The researcher still requires a detailed knowledge about the 'population'. *Opportunistic sampling* relies on selection of those most likely to cooperate with the researcher. Not surprisingly, opportunistic sampling is difficult to replicate. *Snowball sampling* relies on the researcher's knowledge of the situation and the people he or she knows. The researcher contacts people relevant to him or her. Those people then contact people they know, and so on. There is also *theoretical sampling* where the researcher chooses the situation, events or people according to some theoretical purpose (Burgess, 1984: 55–56).

Trade-Offs

There can be trade-offs between different types of validity. Classical laboratory experiments maximize internal validity, because they want to establish causation, but minimize external validity, because laboratory settings are not, by definition, natural settings. Decisions on which method to choose will depend, therefore, on what you want to achieve, as Figure 4.10 shows.

Triangulation

Combining different methods – quantitative and qualitative – to study the same phenomenon has been called *triangulation*. Norman Denzin (1970) said that triangulation involves not only the combination of methods and data, but of theories as well. He said that there are four types of triangulation, including:

1 data triangulation – where the researcher estimates the impact of time, space and different types of interaction (individual, group, and collective) on the data;
2 investigator triangulation, where more than one person examines the same situation;
3 theory triangulation, where alternative or competing theories are used;

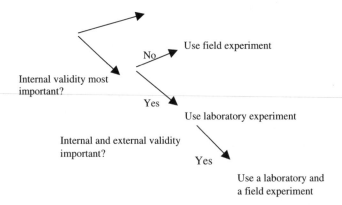

FIGURE 4.10   *Experimental choice based on issues of internal and external validity*

4   methodological triangulation, where the same method is used on different occasions.

Paul Lazarsfeld, the mathematical sociologist, was one of the earliest advocates of combining methods. He and his colleagues attempted to maximize internal and external validity by conducting a natural experiment – a field experiment – in the 1940s and combining that experiment with other methods. Lazarsfeld's study could not be conducted in a laboratory setting because it examined voter intentions and voter behaviour. These phenomena are best studied in their natural setting – a political campaign.

GREAT MEDIA AND POLITICS DETECTIVE STORIES: Using Survey Data. Do media change people's political attitudes? *The People's Choice* (Paul Lazarsfeld)

> Paul F. Lazarsfeld ... virtually created the fields of mathematical sociology, multivariate survey analysis, and the empirical study of both voting behaviour and mass communications
>
> David L. Sills (Rogers, 1994: 244)

Paul Lazarsfeld, a methodologist, joined the Columbia Department of Sociology in 1941. Robert Merton, a theoretician, joined the Department at the same time. Both became famous for developing survey and interview methodology. Merton, the theorist, became expert at interview methodology and first used the words 'focused interview' and 'focused group' and developed the techniques. Lazarsfeld, the methodologist, became expert at media theory and revolutionized media theory and our understanding of how public opinion works.

Lazarsfeld's collaboration with Merton stands in stark constrast to his collaboration with Theodore Adorno. Adorno, the Jewish neo-Marxist Frankfurt School scholar, was interested in the conditions that lead to prejudice and persecution (Adorno had escaped from Nazi Germany). Adorno drew a distinction between 'administrative research', which served government and industry (and which he said described Lazarsfeld's research at the time), and 'critical research', which sought to critique the whole capitalist enterprise and the role of ideology in that enterprise. For Adorno, administrative research could be manipulative and at the service of powerful interests. Critical research was a necessary correction. While Adorno was opposed to quantitative research as 'instrumental' and 'manipulative', he used it himself in his famous study *The Authoritarian Personality*. 'How can one say with assurance that the numerous opinions, attitudes, and values expressed by an individual actually constitute a consistent pattern of organized totality? ... There is no adequate way to proceed other than by actually measuring, in populations, a wide variety of thought contents and determining by means of standard statistical methods which ones go together' (Adorno et al., 1950: 3). Judgements about the significance of the statistics, says Adorno, can only be made 'on the basis of theory' (1950: 3).

The 1940s at Columbia University are a snapshot of the quantitative versus qualitative divide, the study of power as ideology (Adorno) versus the study of influence as the result of many counter-acting variables (Lazarsfeld) and the difference between European and American approaches to the study of communication and sociology. Lazarsfeld, Merton and Adorno were (and remain) a microcosm of the key debates in sociology and methodology.

Adorno and Lazarsfeld shared a common interest: democratization of methods of research – making research methods transparent; and hybridity – making sure that qualitative research informed quantitative research. Lazarsfeld, Berelson and Gaudet's classic work *People's Choice* (1944) is a classic example of hybridity and the creation of a new survey research method to assist with explanatory research.

Methodology and Theory

'We are interested here in all those conditions which determine the political behaviour of people. Briefly, our problem is this: to discover how and why people decided to vote as they did. What were the major influences upon them during the campaign in 1940?' (Lazarsfeld et al., 1944: 1). These opening sentences provide a simple and clear overview of the aims of *People's Choice*. The 1940 presidential election in the United States presented an opportunity to undertake a study of voting intentions in a way not done before.

Previously, voting records were the major material used for analysis of voting behaviour. It enabled the study of the geographical distribution of voting results. University of Chicago researchers in an 'ecological analysis' combined the results of voting with the census data on voters (for example, what the voting patterns might be in predominantly Irish districts). Public opinion polls went a step further by relating political opinion to the characteristics of the individual voter. But these polls were normally conducted with different people and not the same people over time.

Never before had a person's voting intentions been traced through the course of a political campaign. Lazarsfeld used the panel technique – the same set of voters over the period of the political campaign and election – to study voting intentions. Lazarsfeld's theoretical interests were, therefore, twofold – to investigate key influences on voting behaviour and to create a new research method to do so.

Method

Hypotheses and Operationalization

Lazarsfeld had a range of specific research questions he wished to address, such as 'What is the effect of social status upon vote?' 'How are people influenced by the party conventions and the nominations?' 'What role does formal propaganda play?' 'How about the press and the radio?' 'What of the influence of family and friends?' 'Where do issues come in, and how?' 'Why do some people settle their vote early and some late?' 'In short, how do votes develop? Why do people vote as they do? By inference and by direct accounts of the respondents, we shall try to show what influences operated . . .' (Lazarsfeld et al., 1944: 6–7).

Lazarsfeld and his colleagues had specific variables in mind for these research questions, although they held off on premature judgements about which variables had significant influence. Erie County was chosen for the study 'because it was small enough to permit close supervision of the interviewers; because it was relatively free from sectional peculiarities, because it was not dominated by any large urban center, although it did furnish an opportunity to compare rural political opinion with opinion in a small urban center' (Lazarsfeld et al., 1944: 3). Three thousand people were chosen to represent the County. Every fourth house in the County was visited by trained local interviewers, mainly women. Four groups of 600 persons were selected by stratified sampling. Of the four groups, only three were re-interviewed once each. These groups were used as 'control groups' to test the effect that repeated interviewing might have on the panel (Lazarsfeld et al., 1944: 3). The fourth group, the panel, was interviewed once each month from May to November 1940.

Lazarsfeld's interests were multivariate and 'nomothetic'. He was interested in many variables and how they interrelate and influence one another. However, he was also very interested in the 'idiographic' side of the survey research and direct accounts from participants. Whenever a person changed his or her vote intention in any way, from one interview to the next, detailed information was gathered on why he or she had changed. The following narrative on the history of a single voter's intentions over the course of the political campaign gives an idea about how serious Lazarsfeld and his colleagues were in combining aggregated data with individual accounts.

> This young man, undecided in May, voted for Roosevelt in November. But it would be incorrect to assume that at some point during the campaign he simply made up his mind once and for all. Actually, he followed a devious route on his way to the polls. He was a first voter with some high school education and with a slightly better than average socio-economic level. At first he favored Taft for the Republican nomination because he was a fellow resident of Ohio, but on the other side of his indecision was his tendency to vote Democratic 'because my grand-father is affiliated with that party.' This tendency won out in July when he announced that he would vote for Roosevelt to please his grandfather. In August, however, his opposition to the President's stand on conscription gained the upper hand and he came out for Willkie, even though he knew little about him. At this point his vote intention represented a vote against conscription and Roosevelt's pressure for it. At the same time, he generalized this disapproval of conscription into a disapproval of the third term. The following month he changed again: he simply did not know enough about Willkie to cling to him so he reverted to a state of indecision and began to think that he would not vote at all. This attitude persisted throughout the last days of the campaign, when he indicated that the outcome of the election did not make any difference to him. During August and September he believed Willkie would win but later he was undecided on that too, partly because a movie audience had booed the Republican candidate in a newsreel appearance a few days before. But on Election Day, he voted for Roosevelt. He was repelled at the very end of the campaign by what he considered Willkie's begging for votes and he was strongly influenced by fellow workers at the foundry where he was employed. The saga of the formation of his vote illustrates the kinds of data not available before the development of the repeated interview technique. (Lazarsfeld et al., 1944: 5–6)

The quantitative variables of the research in *People's Choice* ranged from social and economic status to religious affiliation and age and various indexes on political predisposition, breadth of opinion, magazine reading, radio listening and general or overall exposure to the campaign, political exposure bias, and agreements with arguments of either side.

Operationalization of 'social and economic status' gives you some idea about how Lazarsfeld and his colleagues went about quantification. Interviewers were trained to assess the homes, possessions, appearance, and manner of speech of members of the sample and to classify them into their proper stratum in the community according to a set quota. 'The people with the best homes, furniture, clothes, etc., i.e., the ones with the most money, would be classed as As; and the people at the other extreme would be Ds. In Erie Country, the quote was approximated in the following distribution: A, 3%; B, 14%; C+ 33%; C−, 30%; and D, 20%' (1944: 17).

Lazarsfeld and his colleagues had simple and complex measurements. For magazine reading, the respondent was asked about several specific articles appearing in current issues of magazines. This index was simply a count of the number of articles on political affairs that the respondent reported reading. In the October interview each respondent was asked whether he or she agreed with eight arguments then current in the political campaign. For example, one of the eight arguments was 'Roosevelt has great personal attractiveness, capacity for hard work, and keen intelligence'. A person who agreed with an argument supporting his or her own side or disagreed with an argument supporting the opposition received a +1 score and a person who disagreed with his or her own argument or agreed with the opposition's argument received a −1 score for each question. Each individual could score between −8 and +8.

Variables

The *People's Choice* study found that variables such as social and economic status, affiliation with 'business' or 'labour' and religious affiliation were good predictors of voters' intentions. Figures 4.11 and 4.12 provide an overview of the results on business and labour affiliation and religious affiliation and their relationship to party choice.

One of Lazarseld's key findings was that mass media appeared to have little influence changing people's minds. It had a reinforcement effect. 'The first thing to say is that some people *were* converted by campaign propaganda but that they were *few* indeed' (Lazarsfeld et al., 1944: 94). An unex-

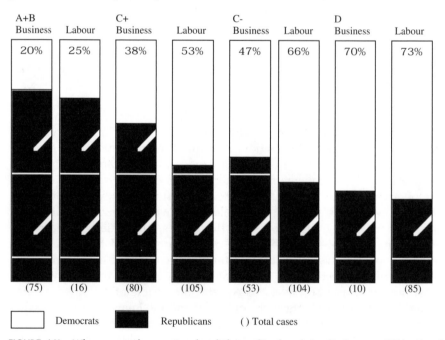

FIGURE 4.11 *Whereas actual occupation does little to refine the relationship between SES level and vote, it makes more difference whether a voter considers himself as belonging to 'business' or 'labour' (adapted from People's Choice)*

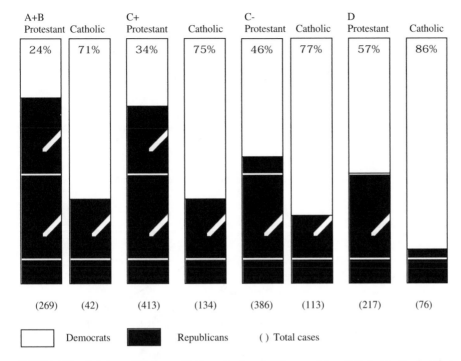

FIGURE 4.12 *Religious affiliation splits the vote sharply. This cannot be attributed to the fact that Catholics in this county are, on average, lower in SES level than Protestants. The relationship between vote and religious affiliation holds true on each SES level.*

pected finding emerged. 'Whenever respondents were asked to report on their recent exposures to campaign communications of all kinds, political discussions were mentioned more frequently than exposure to radio or print' (1944: 150). Those most likely to change their vote in the political campaign 'read and listened least' (1944: 95). Opinion leaders, such as the workers at the foundry in the case of the young man cited earlier, had the most significant influence on outcomes. Mass media did not change behaviour because 'the people who did most of the reading and listening not only read and heard most of their own partisan propaganda but were also most resistant to conversion because of their strong dispositions' (1944: 95). This resistance was also reinforced by the people around them. This recognition of the role of **personal influence** as a mediating factor in mass-media influence led to a complete reconsideration of the nature of mass-media influence. Early models of mass-media influence had assumed a simple cause and effect. Figure 4.13, adapted from *Communication Models* (1981), graphically represents this 'hypodermic' or stimulus–response assumption about mass media. Individuals receive messages and act on them.

Figure 4.14 shows graphically the effect of Lazarsfeld's work on assumptions about the 'receiver'. Lazarsfeld and his colleagues argued that a 'two-step' model of communication was most appropriate to explain mass-media

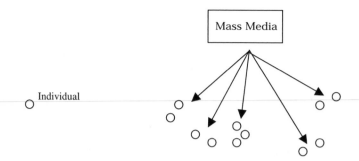

FIGURE 4.13   *One-step model of mass-media influence*

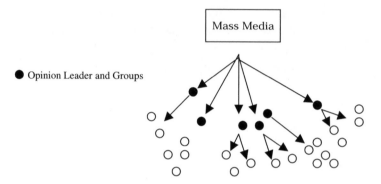

FIGURE 4.14   *Two-step model of mass-media influence*

influence. The vote decisions of 70 per cent of the people, whether or not they expressed an early vote intention, corresponded to the vote tendencies prevailing among groups with social characteristics similar to their own. Social groups, therefore, were a major influence on voting intentions and voting behaviour.

People's Choice demonstrated how sophisticated survey data could get and how the collection of quantitative survey data over time can be complemented with qualitative data. Lazarsfeld was a strong advocate of hybridity – the combining of quantitative with qualitative methods. He concluded that:

1 any phenomenon should be measured with objective observations as well as with introspective reports;
2 case studies should be combined with statistical information;
3 data gathering should be combined with information about the history of what is being studied;
4 data from unobtrusive studies (e.g. observation) should be combined with questionnaire and other self-reported data (Rogers, 1994: 285).

SUMMARY

The ability to recognize what counts as evidence, what counts as clues, is closely related to the sophistication of a research design and its data collection techniques. Umberto Eco's character William of Baskerville got individual clues correct but was mistaken about their overall causal significance. Social science has the same problem. Causality is not easy to establish.

The idea of 'causation' is approached with care by quantitative researchers. Causation and correlation are not the same. Correlation of variables does not establish causation. The idea that causes can be easily established in social science research is wrong. Many of the phenomena a social scientist wishes to study cannot be placed into a laboratory context because (1) it is ethically not possible to manipulate the independent variable or (2) the independent variable in its natural setting cannot be replicated in a laboratory environment.

Experimental methods seek to isolate causes and to maximize internal validity. Experiments intend to explain and have a theoretical purpose in mind. There are two major types of experimental design. Between-subject designs compare groups exposed to the independent variable with control groups that are not exposed. Within-subject designs expose the same groups to the independent variable at different times and the individuals themselves act as a control. Experiments should be used when the researcher is certain that causality is an issue and that the hypothesis is appropriate to experimental research.

Survey methods make possible analysis of large populations and may be exploratory, descriptive or explanatory. 'Populations' are analytically defined by the social scientist. A 'sampling frame' is a list of all members of the researcher's population and can be used to draw a random sample. Questionnaires in surveys use standardized questions. This is an advantage because it is cost effective and relatively quick. However, failure to address the participants' frame of reference can affect the validity of a questionnaire. Social context can affect interpretation of the simplest questions.

All quantitative research methods are subject to bias and error. There is often a trade-off between internal and external validity. Experiments maximize internal validity and surveys maximize external validity. Modern social scientists often combine methods in order to maximize both. Lazarsfeld and his colleagues addressed construct and internal validity by combining qualitative and quantitative understanding of their participants. *People's Choice* refined the panel technique and attempted to isolate the major influences on voting behaviour by examining the same people over time. *People's Choice* is interested in causality but the topic was not appropriate for laboratory research. It is not possible to replicate a presidential campaign in a laboratory setting. Nor is it possible to manipulate the independent variable in the natural setting – for example, to manipulate political campaign propaganda or to change the characteristics of a presidential candidate's personality to see if it made a difference. *People's Choice* did establish a control group to check on interviewer effect and isolated as many of the significant variables as possible.

People's Choice is also an example of a quantitative study that is more 'inductive' than 'deductive', at least in its initial design. *People's Choice* starts with methodology and general research questions, collects data and then works towards theory. Hofstede's study, described in Chapter 3, starts with theory that informed the methodology and the collection of data. Figures 4.15 and 4.16 provide an overview of the differences between the two approaches.

A choice of an inductive or deductive approach depends upon the research topic and the researcher's interests. Both Lazarsfeld and Hofstede were interested in quantitative and qualitative data.

We have investigated many of the issues associated with basic research design and many of the issues associated with operationalization. Now it is time to turn from research design to data analysis. Decisions on research design and methodology affect what counts as evidence – as clues. But there is also the world of statistical analysis that complements research design. The statistical sleuth – the data snooper – can identify

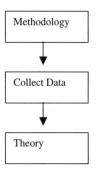

FIGURE 4.15   *Inductive approach*

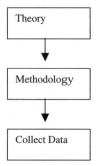

FIGURE 4.16   *Deductive approach*

patterns, regularities and irregularities, in data that are relevant to a study. Numbers tell a story.

MAIN POINTS

- Quantitative methods require detachment of the observer, especially in experimental method where personal involvement can affect the outcomes of the research (unless that effect is accounted for). Personal involvement of the researcher in collecting data, however, is appropriate in a range of research designs.
- There are three main methods of research – case study, survey, and experiment. All three methods can employ different data collection techniques, including questionnaire, interview, content analysis, observation.
- Experimental method involves manipulation of the independent variable and direct observations of the effects of that variable. Between-subject and within-subject designs are the two basic designs in experimental research. Field experiments investigate independent variable(s) in the 'natural' environment.
- The idea of 'causation' captured the popular mind early in the 20th century. Establishing causation, however, involves skill in controlling extraneous variables. Genuine experiments are modest in their conclusions and relate to very specific issues associated with a hypothesis.
- Survey method is appropriate when you cannot observe directly what you want to study. Survey method is particularly appropriate for large populations. Self-administered questionnaires and interview schedules are two of the common techniques of data collection within survey method. Both entail standardization of questions.
- Frame of reference – understanding of the social context in which the survey is to be conducted – is essential to the success of surveys. Frame of reference includes especially the language used by the participants and their understanding of the meanings attached to questions.
- Questions in quantitative questionnaires must be designed with levels of measurement in mind. The level of measurement will affect what kinds of statistical analyses are appropriate. There are two main types of question – closed-ended and open-ended. Closed-ended questions give the participant fixed choices, including a preference not to reply. Open-ended questions may be post-coded by the researcher, where appropriate.
- Multiple-item scales provide a more complex view of underlying attitudes. Summative scales, such as the Likert, are among the most commonly used attitude measures.

- Construct validity and internal validity address problems of operational definition and the relationships between variables. Do our measures really measure what they say they measure?
- External validity addresses problems with sampling. Probability sampling assumes that each member of the defined population has an equal chance of being chosen. Simple random sampling and stratified sampling are two of the most common forms of probability sampling. They maximize external validity.

REVIEW EXERCISES

1 Visit the research ethics site of a university on the internet and download, or examine, their ethics requirements for experimental and survey research. What are the limitations on human experimentation?

2 Create five hypotheses appropriate for an experimental design.

3 Read Stanley Milgram's (1974) *Obedience to Authority: an experimental view* (New York: Harper and Row), or an experiment of interest to you. What were the independent variables?

4 Create a survey design and address the following issues:
   (a) What is the purpose of the survey?
   (b) What is the hypothesis(es)?
   (c) Are operational definitions necessary?
   (d) Create 15 questions relevant to the survey.
   (e) Design a cover letter.

5 Create your own seven-point Likert scale to test a Machiavellian personality.

6 Which sampling technique is most appropriate for the following studies?
   (a) A study to establish the demographic make-up of an audience for local radio.
   (b) A study on teenage use of the internet.
   (c) A study on alcoholism in New York.

REFERENCES

Adorno, T., Frenkel-Brunswick, E., Levinson, D.J. and Nevitt Sanford, R. (1950) *The Authoritarian Personality*. New York: Harper and Brothers.

Aronson, E. and Merrill Carlsmith, J. (1968) 'Experimentation in social psychology', in G. Lindzey and E. Aronson (eds), *The Handbook of Social Psychology*, Volume 2. Reading, Mass.: Addison-Wesley.

Babbie, E. (1986) *The Practice of Social Research*. Belmont, CA: Wadsworth.

Bancroft, G. and Welch, E.H. (1946) 'Recent experience with problems of labor force measurement', *Journal of the American Statistical Association*, 41: 303–12.

Bogardus, E.S. (1925) 'Measuring social distance', *Journal of Applied Sociology*, 9: 299–308.

Bottomore, T.B. and Rubel, M. (eds) (1956) *Karl Marx: Selected Writings in Sociology and Social Philosophy*. New York: McGraw Hill.

Braverman, J. (1974) *Labor and Monopoly Capital: The degradation of work in the twentieth century*. New York: Monthly Review Press.

Burgess, R.G. (1984) *In the Field: an introduction to field research*. London, Unwin Hyman.

Cannell, C. and Kahn, R.L. (1968) 'Interviewing', in G. Lindzey and E. Aronson (eds), *The Handbook of Social Psychology*, Volume 2. Reading, Mass.: Addison-Wesley. pp. 526–95.

Christie, R. and Geis, F.L. (1970) *Studies in Machiavellianism*. New York: Academic Press.

David, F.N. (1962) *Games, Gods and Gambling: The origins and history of probability and statistical ideas from the earliest times to the Newtonian era*. London: Charles Griffin.

Davis, A. (1995) 'The experimental method in psychology', in G.M. Greakwell, S. Hammond and C. Fife-Schaw (eds), *Research Methods in Psychology*. London: Sage.

Denzin, N. (1970) *The Research Act*. Chicago: Aldine.

DeVaus, D.A. (1985) *Surveys in Social Research*. Sydney: Allen and Unwin.

DeVaus, D.A. (1990) *Surveys in Social Research*. Sydney: Allen and Unwin.

Dillman, D.A. (1978) *Mail and Telephone Surveys: the total design method*. New York: Wiley.

Doyle, Arthur Conan (1952) *The Complete Sherlock Holmes*. Garden City, New York: Doubleday.

Eco, U. (1984) *The Name of the Rose*. London: Pan Books.

Fink, A. and Kosecoff, J. (1985) *How to Conduct Surveys: a step-by-step guide*. Newbury Park: Sage.

Hovland, C.I., Lumsdaine, A.A. and Sheffield, F. (1971) 'The effect of presenting "one-sided" versus "both sides" in changing opinions on a controversial topic,' in W. Schramm and D.F. Roberts (eds), *The Process and Effects of Mass Communication*. Urbana, IL: University of Illinois. pp. 467–84.

Hunt, M. (1985) *Profiles of Social Research: The scientific study of human interactions*. New York: Russell Sage Foundation.

Jones, M. (1956) 'TV advertising on its way', *The Australian Monthly*, 23: 25.

Judd, C.M., Smith, E.R. and Kidder, L.H. (1991) *Research Methods in Social Relations*. Forth Worth: Holt, Rinehart and Winston.

Kaplan, R.M. (1987) *Basic Statistics for the Behavioural Sciences*. Allyn and Bacon: Boston.

Lazarsfeld, P.F., Berelson, B. and Gaudet, H. (1944) *The People's Choice: how the voter makes up his mind in a Presidential campaign*. New York: Duell, Sloan and Pearce.

Likert, R. (1932) 'A techique for the measurement of attitudes', *Archives of Psychology*, 140.

McQuail, D. and Windahl, S. (1981) *Communication Models for the Study of Mass Communication*. London: Longman.

Peters, E. (1985) *The Sanctuary Sparrow*. London: Futura.

Rogers, E.M. (1994) *A History of Communication Study*. New York: Free Press.

Sayers, D. (1989) *Whose Body?* Seven Oaks: New English Library.

Schuman, H. and Presser, S. (1977) 'Question wording as an independent variable in survey analysis', *Sociological Methods and Research*, 6: 151–70.

Schwartz, S. (1986) *Classic Studies in Psychology*. Mountain View, CA.: Mayfield.

Shakespeare, W. (1958) *The Complete Works of William Shakespeare*. London: Spring Books.

Simmat, R. (1983) *The Principles and Practice of Marketing*. London: Sir I. Pitman.

Takooshian, H. and Bondinger, H. (1979) *Street Crime in 18 American Cities: a national field experiment.* Paper presented at the annual meeting of the American Sociological Association, Boston, August.

Thurstone, L.L. (1929) 'Theory of attitude measurement', *Psychological Bulletin*, 36: 222–41.

Worsley, P. (1977) *Introducing Sociology*. Harmondsworth: Penguin.

5

'DATA! DATA! DATA!'

Analysing data from the inquiry

'Data! data! data!' he cried impatiently.
'I can't make bricks out of clay'

Sherlock Holmes,
The Adventure of the Copper Beeches

'Data' never comes to the social scientist clean, like cement for bricks. As we found in Chapters 3 and 4, the society a person lives in – and a person's beliefs – can directly affect what counts as a 'clue' and what counts as 'evidence'. Holmes himself was not entirely free from the racial and gender stereotypes of his time. Holmes says, for example, that 'emotional qualities are antagonistic to clear reasoning', but he is equally able to proclaim as fact that 'women are never to be entirely trusted' (*The Sign of Four*). Operational definitions can be affected by the society we live in. But it is wrong to then conclude that we can never retrieve useful quantitative data from the study of psychology or society. Holmes, for all his faults, could see alternative points of view, even if he did not like them: 'if you shift your own point of view a little, you may find it pointing in an equally uncompromising manner to something entirely different' (*The Boscombe Valley Mystery*). Recognition of the problems of validity and making sense of common sense is a good first step in creating a valid and reliable research study. Always ask to see a person's research design; always ask to see their definitions. The same principle holds for exploring statistical data. Always ask for the data! Numbers are not neutral – they form patterns and they tell a story.

LOOKING AT THE CLUES: *The Statistical Sleuth*

Good detective work involves making sense of the clues, making sense of the variables, collected. Hercule Poirot, for instance, sometimes guesses who committed a murder before he has the evidence. 'As I say, I was convinced from the first moment I saw her that Mrs. Tanios was the person I was looking for, but I had absolutely no *proof* of the fact. I had to proceed carefully' (Christie, 1982: 247). Proof of the fact is a part of data analysis in social science research. Proceeding carefully is exactly what you need to do when you start trying to make sense of individual clues.

Why Explore Data?

Some research studies have well-defined hypotheses that are tested by the researcher. Some studies, such as *People's Choice*, have broad research questions that invite exploration. In both cases good data analysts plot their data before they use sophisticated statistical procedures. Graphical displays of data are one of the most important aids in identifying and understanding patterns of data and relationships among variables. Indeed Chambers et al. (1983: 1) go as far as saying that 'there is no statistical tool that is as powerful as a well-chosen graph'.

Over the past two decades a number of new methods for displaying data have been developed that allow for more informative examination of data. Most of these methods belong to a family of techniques known as *exploratory data analysis* (see Tukey, 1977). These tools are particularly appropriate for the statistical sleuth – or the 'data snooper', – as Abelson (1995) aptly put it. The data snooper is an analyst who is vigilant of odd patterns or irregularities in data. These irregularities may suggest that something strange is going on – for example, calculation errors, data entry errors, data not conforming to distributional assumptions or, in more serious cases, data that are fraudulent.

Graphs and plots draw out hidden aspects of the data and relationships among variables that a person may not have anticipated. These 'data-driven discoveries' may spark new investigations previously not considered and may eventually lead to changes in the theories or hypotheses driving the original investigation.

Graphs and plots may complement textual material that in turn may provide a more complete picture of the issue under investigation. Good graphical representations are also good communication. They are easily grasped and therefore easily remembered.

PLOTTING DATA

Stem and Leaf Displays

Variables vary and one of the best ways to see how they vary is to use a stem and leaf display. The stem and leaf display is a quick and easily constructed picture of the shape of a distribution (Tukey, 1977). You do not need a high-powered computer to generate one; if you have a piece of paper and a pencil you can make a stem and leaf display by following some simple steps.

The basic idea of a stem and leaf display is that the digits that make up the numerical values are used in sorting and displaying the numbers. The digit(s) at the beginning of each datum (or leading digits) in a distribution serve to sort the data; the remaining or trailing digits are used to display the data. The leading digits are also referred to as *stems* while the trailing digits are referred to as *leaves*.

A set of very simple rules (based on Moore and McCabe, 1993; Velleman and Hoaglin, 1981) allows us to construct stem and leaf displays:

1 Separate each value into a stem and a leaf. You will need to choose a suitable pair of adjacent digit positions for each datum, say, tens digits and units digits. Usually, stems have as many digits as necessary for displaying the data appropriately for your purpose. On the other hand, each leaf usually has just one digit.
2 Construct a column of all the possible sets of leading digits or stems for the range of values in the distribution in descending order. Draw a vertical line to the right of these stems.
3 For each score, record the leaf on the line labelled by its stem and arrange the leaves in increasing order from left to right.

These rules are applied and illustrated in Example 5.1.

Example 5.1: Stem and leaf display

Performance on an arithmetic test is measured in a small class of children. The scores are as follows:

16   18   14   23   17   13   19   21   16

To construct a simple stem and leaf display we begin by choosing a pair of adjacent digits. In this case a suitable pair of digits would be the tens digit and the units digit. For the value 16 we would split the value 1 (tens digit) and 6 (units digit) where '1' would be the stem and '6' would be the leaf. Now split each value between the two digits. We construct a column for the stems and then write the leaves corresponding to each stem in ascending order.

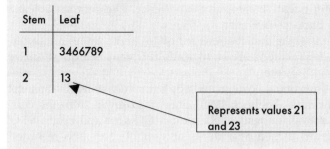

Stem	Leaf
1	3466789
2	13

Represents values 21 and 23

An important feature of stem and leaf displays is that they represent **all** of the data in the distribution. The data are preserved exactly in the 'stem–leaf' arrangement. It is possible to reconstruct the exact values that are represented in the display.

In Example 5.1 we defined the leaves associated with each stem to range from 0–9. Sometimes this range is inappropriate. This is especially the case when you have lots of data. If we had 1,000 observations that ranged between 10 and 30, a stem and leaf display based on stems whose leaves ranged from 0–9 would produce a display with only three very long stems – not a very helpful display. One way to accommodate larger datasets and to obtain a plot that is more meaningful is to 'split' the stem and corresponding leaves into smaller segments. For instance, each stem could have two segments, 0–4 and 5–9. We will use 1• to represent values that lie between 10 and 14, and 1* to represent values that lie between 15 and 19. In other words, the symbols '•' and '*' denote the leaves 0–4 and 5–9 respectively. If we apply these new stems to the data in Example 5.1, we then have a new stem and leaf display that looks as follows:

Stem	Leaf
1•	34
1*	66789
2•	13

You can see that we have a different-looking display. The shape of the distribution has changed. How you split the stem is up to the data snooper. He or she needs to choose a stem that will best identify the salient features of the data under investigation.

Stem and leaf displays can also be used to compare two distributions. Such plots are sometimes referred to as *back-to-back* plots. For example, we may be interested in comparing subjective computer experience using the Subjective Computer Experience Scale among a sample of 10 male and 10 female undergraduate psychology students (Rawstorne et al., 1998). High scores indicate greater negative computer experience. The data in Table 5.1 are followed by the back-to-back plot.

We can clearly see that the distributions for males and females are different. Whether these distributions are statistically different is a question we will answer in the next chapter.

Visual representations of data can provide us with clues when we suspect 'fishiness' in a set of data. Abelson (1995) cites an example from the celebrated Pearce-Pratt studies on tests of clairvoyance (Rhine and Pratt, 1954). An experimenter (Pratt) turned over decks of symbol cards and recorded the sequence, while the clairvoyant (Pearce), who sat in another building, recorded his impressions of what the sequence of symbols had been. A third party then compared the lists and recorded correct matches. There were five possible symbols, so the probability of a match by chance was 20 per cent. However, the reported success rate for matches was 30 per cent – a statistically significant result!! This was quite an extraordinary result, but one

TABLE 5.1   *Example of back-to-back plot*

Males	Females
32	40
45	41
48	60
50	65
55	66
53	55
52	57
45	58
32	67
60	62

Males		Females
22	3	
855	4	01
5320	5	578
0	6	02567

that led critic Hansel (1980) to think about other possible explanations, including fraud! The key observation Hansel made was to note that the success rate was highly variable. Some days yielded upwards of 40 per cent correct, but other days only 15 per cent correct. Why? Inspecting the site on the Duke University campus, Hansel constructed an elaborate hypothesis of fraud. The receiver Pearce, motivated by notoriety as a presumed psychic, cheated. 'On many of the days, he slipped out of the other building as the trials began, hid across the hall from Pratt's office, and stood on a table from which he could see Pratt's symbols through a pair of open transoms. With enough time to copy some or all of them, he left his hiding place and simulated an arrival from the other building. On his symbol sheet, he made sure not to look too perfect, but otherwise produced strong "data". Pratt, his back to the transoms, was an innocent party to the deception' (Abelson, 1995: 82).

A stem and leaf plot of the ESP data got Hansel thinking. The plot is reproduced in Figure 5.1 and represents successful hits per 50 trials.

Hansel found a gap at around the values 10, 11 and 12 – the gap where we would expect a success rate of 20 per cent! The distribution appears to have two modes – a cluster for success days and a cluster for failure days! Could cheating be occurring? Hansel thought so.

Histograms

Stem and leaf displays are useful, but they become cumbersome to construct if you have very large numbers of observations and especially if you do not have access to a computer. One way of dealing with this problem is

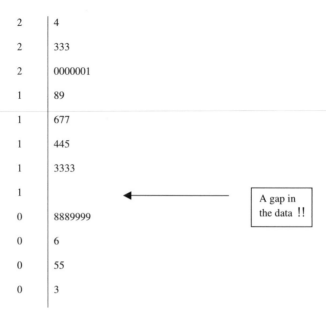

2	4
2	333
2	0000001
1	89
1	677
1	445
1	3333
1	
0	8889999
0	6
0	55
0	3

A gap in the data !!

FIGURE 5.1   A stem and leaf display of ESP data (source: Abelson, 1995: 82)

TABLE 5.2   Frequency distribution table for grouped data

Interval	Midpoint	Frequency	Relative frequency
90–100	95	5	0.05
80–89	85	8	0.08
70–79	75	15	0.15
60–69	65	25	0.25
50–59	55	36	0.36
40–49	45	8	0.08
30–39	35	3	0.03
20–29	25	0	0.00

to divide the range of values into intervals and report the number (or frequency) of observations that fall into each interval. Assume you are a statistics lecturer and you have 100 students enrolled in your introductory statistics class. Assume also that your students have sat their final exam for which they can obtain a mark out of 100. Table 5.2 provides the appropriate layout.

This table is commonly referred to as a *frequency distribution*. Sometimes it is more interesting to examine the *relative* rather than actual frequency of an interval. The relative frequency of an interval is obtained by dividing the frequency of the interval by the total number of observations. This fraction can also be reported as a percentage. Relative frequency distributions are useful if you wish to compare either parts of the same distribution or distributions from two or more groups.

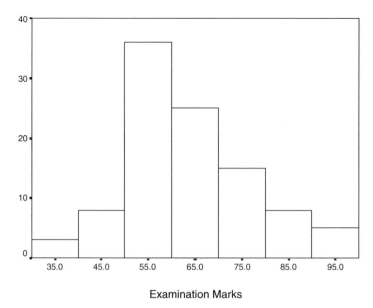

Examination Marks

FIGURE 5.2   *Histogram of hypothetical examination marks*

A *histogram* is a graphical representation of a frequency distribution. The horizontal axis is broken into segments representing the intervals of the scores. The vertical axis represents the frequency of observations. Above each interval on the horizontal axis we draw a bar with height representing the frequency associated with that interval. An example of a histogram of the examination marks data is presented in Figure 5.2.

Boxplots

The *boxplot* is another useful exploratory data analytic technique for representing data visually. Boxplots are useful because the plot depicts the important features of the distribution. A very simple way of examining a distribution is to look at the values that represent:

1   the middle of the distribution (we refer to this value as the *median*);
2   the smallest (minimum) and largest (maximum) value in the distribution;
3   the number that represents the middle value between the median and the minimum value (we will refer to this value as the *first quartile*); and
4   the number that represents the middle value of the scores between the median and the maximum value (we will refer to this value as the *third quartile*).

The term *hinge* is also used to describe a value in the middle of each half of the distribution defined by the median. Hinges are similar to quartiles. The difference between hinges and quartiles is that hinges are defined in terms of the median. They are often located closer to the median than quartiles. The important features of most distributions of scores can be summarized by five values: the minimum and maximum values, and the median and the first and third quartiles. These five values are known as the *five-number summary*. A boxplot is simply a visual representation of the five-number summary (Velleman and Hoaglin, 1981).

The first step is to construct a 'box' whose ends are defined by the first and third quartiles. The length of the box is the difference in the values of the quartiles. The second step is to draw a line within the box represented by the median value. The third step is to draw lines outside the box corresponding to the minimum and maximum values. These lines are also known as *whiskers*. Sometimes the location of the whiskers is defined differently. Some data analysts prefer to define the whiskers of a boxplot in terms of the values that are 1.5 times the difference between the quartiles. If there are scores beyond these modified whisker values, then they are plotted individually. Figure 5.3 gives the anatomy of a boxplot.

We can tell a great deal about a distribution of scores by examining its corresponding boxplot. Consider two hypothetical variables X and Y. A distribution of values for these variables is presented in Table 5.3.

By just 'eye-balling' the data it appears that the values for X are more skewed than the values for Y. The boxplots for the distribution of X and Y are presented in Figure 5.4. Some features of these plots are noteworthy. One observation is that the boxplot for X has only one whisker, an indication that the distribution is skewed. You will also see that the line representing the median is slightly 'off-centre'. This is further evidence that the distribution for X is skewed. On the other hand, you will notice that the median for the distribution of Y is in the middle of the 'box' component of the boxplot, suggesting that the plot is not skewed.

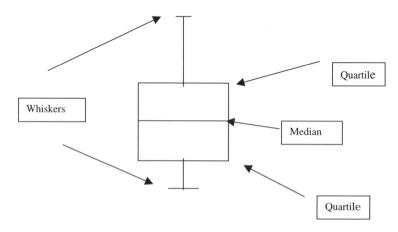

FIGURE 5.3   *The anatomy of a boxplot*

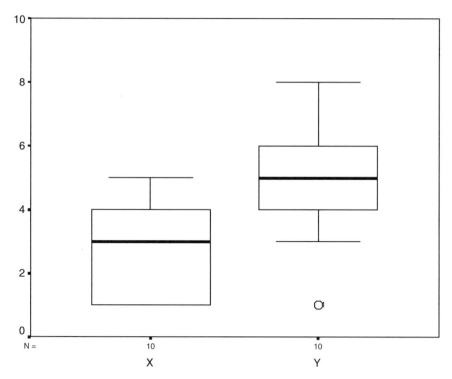

FIGURE 5.4   Boxplots for two hypothetical variables X and Y

TABLE 5.3   Hypothetical data for variables
X and Y

Variable X	Variable Y
1.00	1.00
1.00	3.00
1.00	4.00
2.00	5.00
3.00	6.00
3.00	7.00
4.00	8.00
5.00	5.00
4.00	5.00
3.00	4.00

With a little experience, the data snooper can use boxplots to identify particular features of a distribution. There are two key questions the data snooper can ask when examining a boxplot. First, is one whisker longer than the other whisker? If the answer is yes then this is an indication that the distribution is skewed. With skewed distributions, the bar representing the median will be off-centre. The second question one can ask when investigating a boxplot is whether the 'box' component of the plot is compressed

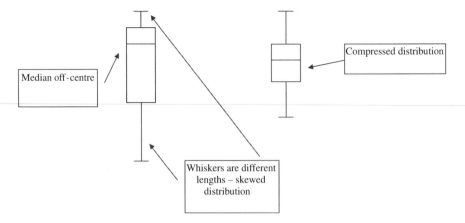

Median off-centre

Compressed distribution

Whiskers are different
lengths – skewed
distribution

FIGURE 5.5   Side-by-side boxplots

or elongated. The 'box' component represents the spread of the middle half of the distribution of values. If the 'box' looks compressed, then the values in the middle half of the distribution are 'close together', falling within a narrow range of values. Figure 5.5 shows these characteristics in two side-by-side boxplots.

Boxplots are useful visual aids. But one should not rely solely on them for understanding a set of data. In some cases, a boxplot can be misleading. For instance, if the data you have just collected are bimodal (have two modes), then a boxplot of those data will not indicate the presence of those modes. In this case, a stem and leaf display would identify the bimodality of the data, and provide the data analyst with a more accurate 'picture' of the data. Boxplots therefore should never be interpreted in isolation.

Tables, Graphs and Figures

'Getting information from a table is like extracting sunlight from a cucumber.' Although this quote from Farquhar and Farquhar (1891) comes at the turn of the 19th century, there are still instances in which the words ring true in the 21st century.

Our knowledge about best practice with tables and graphs has improved since Farquhar and Farquhar's day. Wainer (1992) found, from an analysis of the use of tables and graphs to represent measurements, that they are best used for three main purposes:

1   Tables and graphs can be used to identify and to extract single bits of information; for example, what types of crimes were committed in Sydney, Australia in 1999?
2   Tables and graphs can be used for trends, clusters or groupings; for example, have the types of crimes in Sydney changed during 1995 to 1999?

3   Tables and graphs can be used to make group comparisons; for example, we can ask the question, which crime is most frequent? Are the types of crimes committed in Sydney different from those in London?

Tables and graphs represent a convenient and an effective way of summarizing information. A good table should enable the reader to understand at a glance information that would be difficult to grasp if presented in the text. A good table is simple and conveys information concisely.

The components of tables and graphs have also been the subject of study. Sternberg (1977) said that a table has several key components:

1   Tables should be numbered. It is important to be able to identify a table accurately when it is being discussed in the text,
2   Tables should be labelled appropriately and concisely. The title should be unambiguous and understandable without reference to the text,
3   Tables usually contain columns. These columns should be clearly labelled.

Sternberg identified four types of column headings. The first type of heading is a stubhead. This column is typically located on the left of the table and usually lists the independent variables in the study. The second type of heading is called a boxhead; these are the headings at the top of a table. Boxheads may cover more than one column. These subdivisions of a boxhead are referred to as column heads. The final type of heading that Sternberg identified was a spanner head. Spanner heads cover the entire body of a table. Some of these heading types are illustrated in the example in Table 5.4, from Ho and Zemaitis (1981: 24).

The body of the table can contain both numerical and written content. In the case of numerical content, the level of precision should be no more than the data justify. Tables can also have footnotes. These should be informative and concise.

Figures also enable the researcher to present information concisely. Figures are useful because we can see at a glance conspicuous features of the data. However, figures and graphs do have one important disadvantage – they do not necessarily reveal precise values. Tables, on the other hand, are precise and concise tools for conveying data and statistical information (Sternberg, 1977).

Figures and graphs, like tables, should be titled. The title (also referred to as the figure caption) should describe clearly and concisely what the graph is reputed to demonstrate. The reader should be able to understand what the figure or graph is about from the title without needing to refer to the text. Figures should also be numbered. We usually use Arabic numbers to refer to figures (Sternberg, 1977).

Finally, the text should not reproduce material presented in tables and graphs. Obviously, it is important to discuss graphs and tables. They are, after all, summaries (visual summaries in the case of graphs) of data and

TABLE 5.4   *The anatomy of a table (used by permission)*

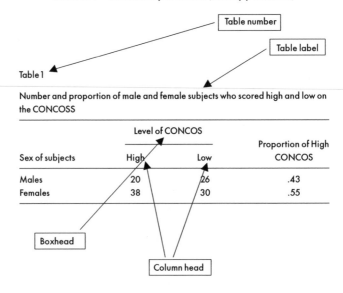

information, and therefore need to be explained and elaborated in the text. However, it is not good practice to replicate the content of a table or graph in the text.

Does a Picture Always Paint a Thousand Words? Some issues with representing data in graphical and tabular form

Although graphs and tables can be effective and efficient ways of conveying and summarizing large amounts of information, there are occasions where these tools can be used to mislead the inexperienced statistical sleuth.

One common trick used by researchers (and market researchers and advertisers in particular) is manipulating the scale intervals on a graph in order to exaggerate the result or finding. Let us assume that we have surveyed the residents of a large Australian city to examine the preferred telecommunications carrier. The researchers find that 53 per cent of respondents preferred Carrier A while 47 per cent of respondents preferred Carrier B. We can present these findings in a histogram as shown in Figure 5.6.

An inspection of this graph suggests that, although there is a difference between preferences, this difference is small. Now consider the same data presented in a somewhat different manner in Figure 5.7.

By changing the scale values in the vertical axis we have exaggerated the difference between the preference for the two carriers. Note that in the second figure we start the values on the vertical axis with 44, not 0 as is the case in Figure 5.6. The experienced data snooper will check the values on the scales depicted in graphs. As a rule of thumb, the scale values on the vertical axis should begin with 0.

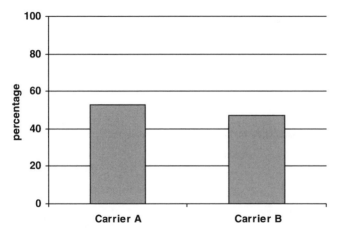

FIGURE 5.6   *Preference for telecommunications carrier*

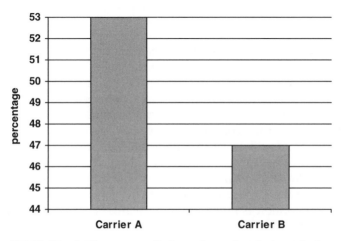

FIGURE 5.7   *A different way to display preference for telecommunications carrier*

The manipulation of information in a table or graph is not always intended to mislead the reader. Abelson (1995) provides an example of data manipulation or 'reframing' (quite legitimately) that assists the articulation of the results. Abelson cites a study by Beall (1994) that examines the stereotype of women as more emotionally expressive than men. Abelson notes that Beall presented male and female participants with a number of vignettes. These vignettes depicted relatively simple social behaviours such as touching someone's arm. Each vignette involved either a hypothetical man or woman engaging in the behaviour. The behaviours were held constant in these two versions. Each participant was asked to report the intensity of the emotion using a seven-point scale. The data in Table 5.5 represent the mean intensity rating averaged over the vignette completed by participants.

TABLE 5.5   Mean ratings of intensity of emotion

	Gender of story character	
Gender of subject	Male	Female
Male	4.52	4.20
Female	4.46	4.66
Column means	4.49	4.43

Source: Abelson, 1995: 116

TABLE 5.6   Reframed data: mean ratings of intensity of emotion

	Gender of story character relative to participant	
Gender of subject	Male	Female
Male	4.52	4.20
Female	4.66	4.46
Column means	4.59	4.33

Source: Abelson, 1995

The means in this table tell us that female participants attribute more emotional intensity to the behaviours than do males, but females do not attribute more emotional intensity when the characters are male. As Abelson notes, trying to understand the interaction between gender of the participant and gender of the character is not straightforward in terms of the original labelling of the columns in Table 5.5. A simple rearranging or reframing of the data will assist in aiding the interpretation of the inter- action. Table 5.6 presents the reframed data. Note that the columns now represent the gender of the character relative to the subject – is the gender of the character either the same as or opposite to the gender of the participant?

Now the interpretation is more straightforward: Females attribute more emotional intensity to characters that are of the same gender and opposite gender than do males, but both males and females attribute more emotional intensity to characters of their own gender (Abelson, 1995: 116). Reframing the data has not tampered with its integrity. It has simply aided the reader in understanding the point that the author wishes to make. It's a matter of looking at the clues from a different angle or perspective.

USING SPSS AND EXCEL TO PLOT DATA:
Accounting for Tastes dataset

We will use a real dataset to show how SPSS and Excel, statistical and spreadsheet software, can be used to plot and describe data. The SPSS dataset, *tastes.sav,* has been taken by the authors from Bennett, Emmison and Frow's comprehensive 1995 survey on the everyday culture of Australians. The innovative survey is reported in *Accounting for Tastes:*

Australian Everyday Culture. Like our other case studies, it is an excellent example of care taken in theory, the relationship between quantitative and qualitative, operationalization and sampling.

Methodology and Operationalization

Bennett et al. (1999) wanted to find out about the relationship between social class and culture. Do countries like Australia have a ruling class that directly affects cultural choice (like going to the theatre, listening to pop music)? Is there a 'single powerful and universally binding scale of cultural legitimacy which produces effects'? (1999: 269).

Accounting for Tastes is both a theoretical critique of Pierre Bourdieu's ideas of social class and a presentation of their own ideas of 'regimes of value' (1999: 258–264). According to Bennett et al., regimes of value are templates which structure cultural preferences. The templates might not in all cases be explicitly set out: 'but they are expressed and refined at every level of cultural legislation, from literary and film criticism, to discussion at work about last night's television programs, to transient comments about someone's good or bad taste in jewellery or in souped-up cars or in colour schemes for the house' (1999: 259–260). Regimes of value can be stable over time because they are grounded in administrative, economic, technological, and legal infrastructures. 'They are never simply expressive of, and never simply reflect, a class structure, or the ethos of an age cohort or a gender or a structure of sexual preference' (1999: 260).

To operationalize the Australian Everyday Cultures Project (AECP) class model, Bennett and his colleagues collected information about their participants' current occupation to determine their employment status as well as managerial or supervisory status. 'On these initial filters we superimposed a measure of the occupation's skill level based on the groups of the Australian Standard Classification of Occupations (ASCO) devised by the Australian Bureau of Statistics' (1999: 18). The resulting 'class model' consisted of nine categories: Never employed, employers, self-employed, managers, professionals, para-professionals, supervisors, sales and clerical workers, and manual workers.

'Cultural tastes' were defined by everything that the AECP could conceive as 'culture': 'including home-based leisure activities, fashion, the ownership of cars and electronic equipment, eating habits, friendships, holidays, outdoor activities, gambling, sport, reading, artistic pursuits, watching television, cinema-going, and the use of libraries, museums and art galleries' (1999: 2).

The sampling frame for the AECP survey was based on the August 1994 Australian Electoral Roll. 'A total of 5000 non-institutionalized adults were obtained by firstly stratifying by state and territory and then applying systematic random sampling within these strata' (1999: 270). Of 5,000 questionnaires a total of 500 were returned undelivered; 450 were returned

TABLE 5.7   Accounting for tastes: comparison of stratified sample with official stastistics

Australian State/Territory	1995 Everyday Culture Survey	1994 Australian Bureau of Statistics estimates
Northern Territory (19)	0.7	1.0
Australian Capital Territory (51)	1.9	1.7
Tasmania (72)	2.6	2.6
Western Australia (246)	8.9	9.6
South Australia (253)	9.2	8.2
Queensland (529)	19.2	18.0
New South Wales (867)	31.5	33.9
Victoria (719)	26.1	25.0
N = 2,756	100.0	100.0

as refusals, with a total of 2,756 usable returns, making a response rate of 61.9 per cent. Table 5.7 shows the stratified sample and the official statistics.

Bennett et al. (1999) also conducted a major pilot in Brisbane and associated areas before conducting the survey. This included extensive qualitative focus groups in order to explore frame of reference. Data from these groups are represented in the study, providing an ethnographic component to the study. Bennett and his colleagues acknowledged the limitations that definition of constructs may place on their findings:

> The categories that organise our survey are constructs, artifices of method which frames the questions in a certain way, chooses a particular form of the independent variables, weights the data to conform to the national census figures, and subjects them to complex statistical manipulations (each with its inbuilt assumptions) to produce the 'findings' which then form the raw material for theoretical interpretation. (1999: 15)

While *Accounting for Tastes* had theoretical reservations regarding quantitative survey methods, it argued that these problems related mainly to how the results of such methods are presented, rather than the unsuitability of quantitative methods *per se*. 'We said earlier that our interest in such methods was prompted partly by a wish to subject cultural studies to a disciplined form of engagement with "the real". The danger, though, is that if interpreted in the light of the positivist assumptions which often accompany them, the results of quantitative methodologies can often be mistaken for reality itself' (1999: 15). Here we have echoes of both Hoftstede and Lazarsfeld.

Working with SPSS

The dataset for *Accounting for Tastes* is available through the Australian National University Social Sciences Data Archive (http://ssda.anu. edu.au/). The description below, provided through the archive, provides an overview of the dataset and the study itself. Many scholars send their datasets to data archives in order to provide other researchers with access to the raw data. There is normally a small fee for ordering the dataset and specific permissions required for using those datasets.

Social Science Data Archives
The Australian National University

Research Topic (Abstract)
The Australian Everyday Consumption project represents the first ever study of Australians' cultural consumption. The study aims to delineate the cultural activities of Australians and their relationship to social class. The survey covers a broad range of cultural pursuits, and variables include the books, newspapers and magazines people read; the film and television programs they watch; the types of cars they drive and possession of other consumer durables; their musical interests; the suburbs they live in; their homes and levels of home ownership; whether they gamble; their hobbies; whether they play and/or watch sport; membership of clubs; what they eat; their pets; how often they attend galleries, concerts and/or the theatre; the clothes they wear; their families and friends; working conditions and working hours; comparisons with spouse and parents; personal and household financial details; religious beliefs and practices; and their attitudes towards societal classes, culture, politics and government, finance and the economy, trade unions, gender and employment, and Aboriginal land rights. Background variables include respondents age, sex, marital status, level of education, country of birth, work status, income and occupation.

Subject Terms
Accommodation; Arts; Assimilation (cultural); Attitudes; Broadcasting; Careers; Clothing; Clubs; Community involvement; Diet; Education; Employment; Ethnic groups; Family; Films; Food; Gambling; Human relations; Income; Leisure; Living standards; Mass media; Motor cars; Music; Newspapers; Performing arts; Politics; Radio; Radio programmes; Reading; Religion; Social classes; Social responsibility; Sports; Television; Television programmes; Travel; Values; Working conditions; Working hours.

Kind of Data
Survey

Time Dimensions
cross-sectional (one-time) study

Definition of Total Universe (Universe Sampled)
All non-institutionalised Australian adults, aged 18 years and over who were on the July 1994 Commonwealth Electoral Roll.

Sampling Procedures
Stratified random sample

Number of Units (Cases)
number of units in original sample: 5,000
number of losses: 2,244
number of replacements: 0
number of cases (unweighted): 2,756

Dates of Data Collection
first date of data collection: November 1994
last date of data collection: March 1995

Method of Data Collection
self-completion (mail out, mail back)

Dimensions of Dataset
number of cases: 2,756.
number of variables per case: 633

Accessibility
A copy of the User Undertaking Form must be signed before data may be accessed.

The datafile *tastes.sav* is in SPSS format. SPSS is one of the most commonly used statistical packages in the social sciences. We will use Version 9.0 of SPSS to show how histograms, stem and leaf displays and boxplots are obtained from SPSS. *The Statistical Inquirer,* multimedia courseware provided with this text, provides introductory lessons in descriptive statistics. The courseware also provides brief, dynamic, exercises on the functions of SPSS. The exercises use a real dataset from the doctoral work of Patrick Rawstorne at the University of Wollongong. This dataset is available as an SPSS file for practice in SPSS.

Once you have opened a data file in SPSS, such as the *Accounting for Tastes tastes.sav* file that we are using here, the data editor in SPSS will look like this.

tastes - SPSS for Windows Data Editor

File Edit View Data Transform Analyze Graphs Utilities Window Help

1:housinc   75000

	tertqual	school	jobinc	housinc	gold
1	1.00	2.00	75000.00	75000.00	1.00
2	4.00	1.00	7500.00	23000.00	4.00
3	1.00	1.00	55000.00	55000.00	2.00
4	4.00	1.00	7500.00	13500.00	-2.00
5	4.00	1.00	36000.00	29000.00	2.00
6	1.00	2.00	45000.00	75000.00	2.00
7	4.00	1.00	10500.00	13500.00	7.00
8	4.00	1.00	21000.00	45000.00	2.00

Let's consider the variable 'housinc', annual household income. We may be interested in exploring the distribution of annual household incomes. In this chapter we have looked at histograms, stem and leaf displays and boxplots as ways of representing data visually. There are a number of ways of using SPSS to construct these plots. One way is to use the *Explore* option. Select *Descriptive Statistics* from the *Analyze* menu. Choose the *Explore* option from *Descriptive Statistics*.

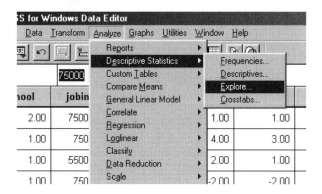

Once you have selected *Explore*, the following dialog box will appear.

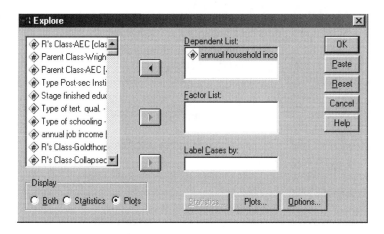

Select the variable you wish to analyse, in this case 'housinc', and move it to the *Dependent List* window by clicking on the uppermost arrow button. Select the *Plots* display button located in the lower left-hand corner of the dialog box.

The next step is to select the types of plots you wish to construct. This is done by clicking on the *Plots* button located on the lower right-hand corner of the window. [Note that you also have the option of comparing boxplots. You could, for example, include a grouping variable in the *Factor List* window. This would allow you to draw boxplots for each level of the grouping variable, such as gender.] The following window should appear.

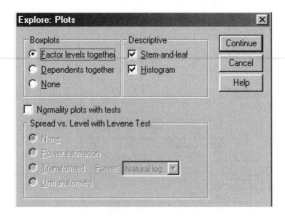

Ensure that the *Histogram* option is checked. The *boxplot* and *stem and leaf* display options are default selections. Then click *Continue* and OK. This will generate the output.

Here is the stem and leaf display output associated with the same data.

Frequency	Stem & Leaf
106.00	0 . 00000000000013
106.00	0 . 555777777777777
190.00	1 . 0000000000003333333333333333
174.00	1 . 66666666666666666999999999
162.00	2 . 111111111111133333333333
286.00	2 . 55555555555555599999999999999999999999999
.00	3 .
216.00	3 . 666666666666666666666666666666
.00	4 .
265.00	4 . 5555555555555555555555555555555555555
.00	5 .
222.00	5 . 5555555555555555555555555555555
.00	6 .
192.00	6 . 55555555555555555555555555
.00	7 .
134.00	7 . 55555555555555555
.00	8 .
62.00	8 . 555555555
.00	9 .
57.00	9 . 55555555
111.00	Extremes (>= 110000)

Stem width: 10000.00
Each leaf: 7 case(s)

The boxplot output summarizes the distribution:

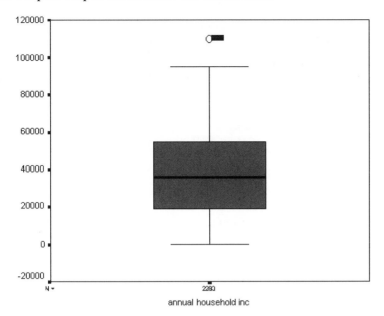

We can see from these displays that the data on household income are slightly skewed. The histogram and stem and leaf representations are asymmetrical; most of the values are between $10,000 and $45,000. From the boxplot display we see that the whiskers are of different lengths and the median is just slightly off-centre – clues that the data may be skewed. The boxplot display also indicates the presence of possible extreme values (annual household incomes of $110,000).

Histograms and boxplots can also be constructed by selecting *Histogram* or *Boxplot* from the *Graphs* menu.

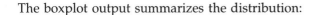

If you select the *Boxplot* option, the following dialog box appears.

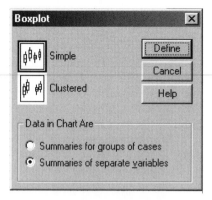

Ensure that you have selected *Summaries of separate variables* by clicking on it. Click on *Define* to obtain the next dialog box.

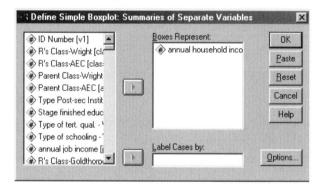

We will select the variable 'housinc', labelled annual household income, and move it to the *Boxes Represent* window by clicking on the arrow button. Click on *OK* to generate the output.

If you select *Histogram* from the *Graphs* option you will see the following dialog box.

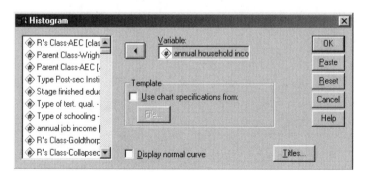

Select the variable from the variable list and move it to the *Variable* window by clicking on the arrow button. Click on *OK* to generate the histogram.

Working with Excel

There are alternative software packages that enable you to create histograms, stem and leaf displays and boxplots. Microsoft's Windows 97 version of Excel is not a statistical package. None the less, it provides a number of very useful data manipulation and data analytic tools. Excel does not provide a menu option that will allow you to construct stem and leaf displays or boxplots. However, it is possible to write macros in Excel that would allow you to construct these plots.

There are a number of ways to construct a histogram using Excel. One way is to make use of the data analysis tools available in the *Analysis ToolPak*. The data analysis procedures are available from the *Tools* menu. The following example uses the 'housinc' variable from the *tastes.sav* data file.

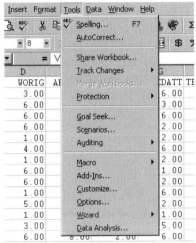

From this menu you can select the *Data Analysis* option and access the following dialog box. The Data Analysis dialog box lists a number of statistical procedures, including the option for constructing a histogram.

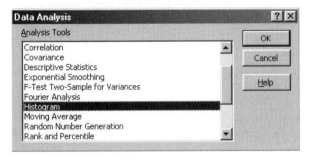

Select *Histogram* and click *OK*. You should now have the next dialog box.

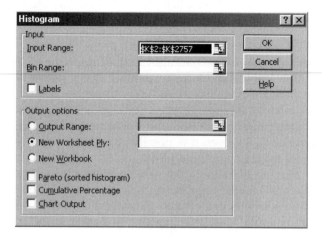

In this box we include the cell range that includes the data we wish to analyse. You select this range by simply clicking on the first cell (not the cell containing the variable label) of the column containing the data and then clicking on the last cell. Click *OK*. This procedure will generate a frequency distribution on a separate Excel worksheet. You can then use the chart wizard to construct a graph of this frequency distribution.

DESCRIBING DATA

Numerical Summaries: What are they and why are they important?

We have looked at ways of graphically representing a set of numerical values for a particular variable. We can use these techniques to compare sets of values or distributions. However, there is a problem associated with using some graphical techniques to compare distributions. The problem is related to the fact that plots such as stem and leaf displays represent all the data at an individual level. It is important to be able to *summarize* the main features or properties of a distribution of scores. The experienced data snooper responds to the request 'Give me the facts' not by taking short cuts but by summarizing the facts in a meaningful way and without substantial loss of information.

Most distributions have three important features, namely, the *shape* of the distribution, the *location* or central tendency of the distribution and the *spread* of scores in that distribution. For a particular distribution it is possible to derive measures or indices for these distributional characteristics.

Describing Location or Centrality

Some Notation

To assist us in defining some indices of location and spread, it is useful to use some mathematical notation. Any kind of mathematical notation is enough to send some people into fits of panic. For those of you who are 'notation phobic', remember that mathematics is just another language that we can learn – admittedly a very specialized language, but parts of it are easy to learn. The game is afoot!!

Assume we are measuring a variable – the number of standard drinks consumed by Australian men aged between 20 and 21. For illustrative purposes let us also assume that we have data for five men. The values are 3 5 2 4 4 respectively. We can use the letter X to represent the variable of interest, in this case, number of standard drinks consumed by Australian men aged between 20 and 21. In this example, the variable takes on five values. Let the individual values be represented by $x_1, x_2, x_3, x_4,$ and x_5 respectively. The subscript identifies a particular individual. That is, x_1 represents the value for person 1 (the value 3), x_2 represents the value for person 2 (the value 5), and so on. If we had n individuals then the nth value for the variable X would be represented as x_n, and the value for the ith individual would be represented by x_i.

In defining some numerical summaries we want to add up or sum values. The operation of summing values is abbreviated or represented by Σ, the Greek letter upper-case sigma. The operation of summing n values, $x_1, x_2, \ldots, x_n$, that is $x_1 + x_2 + \ldots + x_n$, can be represented as Σx_i.

The most used and familiar measure of centrality is the *arithmetic mean* or average. Computing the mean is quite simple. You simply add up the values and divide by the number of values that you have. If we have n values, $x_1, x_2, \ldots, x_n$, then the mean, M, is represented algebraically as:

$$M = (x_1 + x_2 + \ldots + x_n)/n$$

Another important measure of centrality is the *median*. We introduced this index when we discussed boxplots earlier. You will recall that the median is defined as the point at or below which 50 per cent of the values fall. If we were to rank-order our data from lowest to highest values, then the median is the middle value in the rank order. Therefore, the median may be thought of as the 'typical' value in a set of data.

Assuming we have n values, we can use the formula $(n + 1)/2$ to calculate the rank position of the median. If we have an odd number of values, this formula will give an integer value for the rank position. However, if we have an even number of values, the rank will not be integer. In this case we define the median as the rank of the two middle values in the distribution.

Example 5.2: Calculating the median of odd and even numbered distributions

The following numbers are measures of diastolic blood pressure obtained from five men in an experiment on reactions to the movie *The Hound of the Baskervilles*:

$$72 \ 88 \ 90 \ 84 \ 86$$

To calculate the median we first rank-order the scores:

$$72 \ 84 \ 86 \ 88 \ 90$$

Using formula $(n+1)/2$ we find that the rank position of the median is $(5+1)/2 = 3$. The third value in the set of values is 86.

We also obtain the diastolic blood pressure for a sixth man, with a value of 100. Then the rank position of the median is $(6+1)/2 = 3.5$. The median lies between the third and fourth values of our ordered set, namely 86 and 88. The median in this case is the average of these two values, namely $(86+88)/2 = 87$. Note that the value of the median is not actually in our set of values.

A median can be found for data that are usually interval in nature, although you could find the median ordinal data. However, we generally do not calculate the median for categorical or nominal-level data since these classes of measurement are not ordered.

A third measure of central tendency is the *mode*. It is probably the most obvious measure of location. The mode is simply the most frequently occurring value in a distribution. This definition allows for the possibility of more than one mode for a distribution. This is one reason why the mode is not particularly useful as a measure of centrality and therefore not generally reported.

Mean vs. Median (When is the evidence not contaminated?)

Although both are measures of centrality the mean and median do not measure the same thing. Consider the following scenario. You are asked by a close and dear friend to help him purchase a home. He is returning to your suburb after working interstate for a number of years. Being a good friend you decide to help him out by inquiring about home prices in your suburb. You visit the local professor in real estate, Professor Moriarty, and are told that the average home prices in your area have risen from $200,000 to $300,000 in the past two years. This seems like excellent news for your friend. Or is it? Is the average home price the best indicator of values in your area? Or is this statistic 'contaminated'?

The mean or average is not always the best indicator of the 'typical' value in a set of data. Consider the following home prices in a quiet cul-de-sac:

$$\$150,000 \quad \$160,000 \quad \$170,000 \quad \$170,000 \quad \$180,000$$

The average of these values is $166,000; the median value is $170,000. Now let us assume that the home valued at $150,000 is sold, demolished and a new home built in its place, valued at $300,000. What effect does this have on the mean and median values? The median value is still $170,000 but the mean value has rise to $196,000! Does the mean still represent the typical home price in the street? You can see that having an atypical or extreme value in a set of data affects the mean value. In fact you can make the mean as large as you like simply by increasing the value of just one value in the batch! On the other hand, the median is unaffected by or *resistant* to these extreme values. That is, the median is a *resistant measure*.

Will you ask Professor Moriarty for more clues? What would the good data snooper ask for?

Describing Variability

An important characteristic of a set or distribution of values is the way those values vary from each other, the spread or variability of the distribution. At times it is more important to consider how scores vary than to describe the typical value in a distribution of scores. For example, the median annual incomes of two groups of individuals may be the same, but, for one group, the distribution of scores may have some extreme values, indicating extremes in relative incomes (and wealth, if wealth is operationalized as annual income!).

One way to describe the variability of scores in a distribution is to plot those scores. But are there summary measures or indices of variability that we can use?

A very simple measure of spread is the *range*. The range is defined as the difference between the largest and smallest values in the distribution. Consider two sets of scores:

$$\text{Set 1:} \quad 2 \quad 6 \quad 7 \quad 8 \quad 10 \quad 11$$

$$\text{Set 2:} \quad 1 \quad 1 \quad 1 \quad 2 \quad 3 \quad 3$$

The range for Set 1 is $11 - 2 = 9$, while the range for Set 2 is $3 - 1 = 2$. You can see that Set 1 has a larger range than Set 2, indicating that the spread of scores is greater for Set 1 than Set 2. However, the range is not a resistant measure of spread. Let's say Set 2 consisted of the following values:

$$\text{Set 2:} \quad 1 \quad 1 \quad 1 \quad 2 \quad 3 \quad 10$$

The range is now is $10 - 1 = 9$, the same as for Set 1. But the spread of scores for each distribution is quite different!

We can describe the spread of a distribution in terms of percentiles. A *percentile* corresponds to a value in a distribution such that a certain percentage of the distribution falls above or below it. The median, for example, is the 50th percentile, since 50 per cent of the values in a distribution fall above the median, and 50 per cent fall below it.

We defined two other important percentiles when we discussed boxplots. Quartiles are percentiles; the *first quartile* (abbreviated Q_1) is the 25th percentile, and the *third quartile* (Q_3) is the 75th percentile. The quartiles are quite simple to calculate. We first need to rank-order our observations. We then locate the median. The first quartile is the median of those observations that lie below the median. The third quartile is the median of those values above the median. Imagine a piece of paper representing the set of observations. If you fold the paper into two equal halves, the fold represents the median. If you fold the paper again so that you have four equal quarters, the first and third fold marks represent the first and third quartiles.

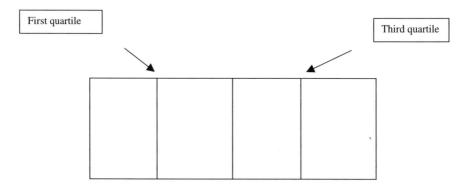

A very simple and useful measure of spread is the distance between the quartiles. This measure is known as the *interquartile range* (*IQR*). Symbolically,

$$IQR = Q_3 - Q_1$$

You will recall that it corresponds to the edges of the 'box' in a boxplot. An important feature of the quartiles and the *IQR* is that they are resistant measures.

The *IQR* can also be used to identify extreme values in a set of observations. One commonly used rule is to define extreme values or outliers as those values that lie at least 1.5 times the value of the *IQR* ($1.5 \times IQR$) below the first quartile or above the third quartile.

Perhaps the most commonly used measure of spread is the *variance* (and the associated measure of *standard deviation*). These measures are defined in terms of variation about the mean as the measure of location. These measures, therefore, are not resistant, yet they are extremely common in social science research.

The logic behind variance as a measure of spread goes as follows: Let's define the mean (M) as the measure of centrality of a set of n observations (x_i). Each observation deviates from the mean by a certain amount ($x_i - M$). Now one possible measure of spread would be to add up all possible deviations. However, some observations will lie below the mean, and therefore, $x_i - M$ will be negative; some observations will fall above the mean and $x_i - M$ will be positive. In fact the sum of these deviations, $x_i - M$, will always be 0. A way around this problem is to square the deviations before summing them. The variance is computed by taking the sum of squared deviations and dividing this sum by $n - 1$. The variance can be interpreted as an average squared deviation. We will use the symbol s^2 to represent the variance. Algebraically, s^2 is:

$$s^2 = 1/(n-1)[(x_1 - M)^2 + (x_2 - M)^2 + \ldots + (x_n - M)^2]$$

The variance has one disadvantage as a measure of spread. Let's say you are measuring weight in kg, then the variance will be measured in squared kg, since we are computing squared deviations. To return the variance to the same units of measurement as the original values, we take the square root of the variance. We call this new index the *standard deviation*, represented symbolically as *s*.

Example 5.3: Calculating the variance of a set of values

Famous psychologist Prof. Loshonski has constructed a new measure to assess the degree to which people are susceptible to deception. The measure generates a score ranging from 1 to 20, where 1 means 'not susceptible at all' and 20 means 'extremely susceptible'. Prof. Loshonski obtains scores from five people. Their scores are 4, 6, 8, 10, 12, respectively. To calculate the variance of these scores we begin by computing the mean.

$$M = (4 + 6 + 8 + 10 + 12)/5 = 40/5 = 8$$

Next we calculate the deviation scores, square them and sum up. These computations are presented in the following table:

x_i	$x_i - M$	$(x_i - M)^2$
4	$4 - 8 = -4$	$(-4)^2 = 16$
6	$6 - 8 = -2$	$(-2)^2 = 4$
8	$8 - 8 = 0$	$(0)^2 = 0$
10	$10 - 8 = 2$	$(2)^2 = 4$
12	$12 - 8 = 4$	$(4)^2 = 16$
	$(x_i - M) = 0$	$(xi - M)^2 = 40$

$$s^2 = 1/(n-1)[(x_1 - M)^2 + (x_2 - M)^2 + \ldots + (x_n - M)^2]$$
$$= 1/(n-1)[16 + 4 + 0 + 4 + 16]$$
$$= 1/(5-1)[40]$$
$$= 40/10$$
$$= 10$$

The variance of the five scores is 10. The standard deviation is the square root of 10 which is 3.16.

We have already noted that the standard deviation is not a resistant measure of spread. If the distribution is skewed, the standard deviation will not be a good measure of spread. So why use it? One reason is that the standard deviation plays an important role in mathematical statistics, in particular in its role in the normal distribution. We will examine this role in the next chapter. But for now it is important to note that the good statistical sleuth will be cautious about interpreting indices in isolation. You need to look at all the facts, not just one bit of evidence. You cannot interpret an index or measure like the standard deviation without asking 'Show me the data!! Show the me data!!'. Indices such as the standard deviation need to be interpreted in the context of the distribution they are based on.

USING SPSS AND EXCEL TO DESCRIBE DATA

Working with SPSS

The *Explore* option in SPSS allows the researcher to construct histograms, stem and leaf displays and boxplots for a set of values. This option, however, can also be used to generate all of the descriptive statistics we have discussed in this chapter. Let's consider again the variable 'housinc' for the *tastes.sav* data file.

Recall that we access the *Explore* option by going to the *Analyze* menu and then selecting *Descriptive Statistics*. The following dialog box should appear.

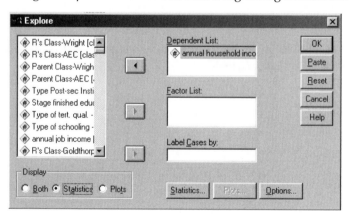

Select the variable of interest, in this case 'housinc', and move it to the *Dependent List*. Select *Statistics* from the *Display* option located in the lower left-hand corner of the dialog box. Clicking on the *Statistics* button located in the lower right-hand corner of the dialog box will bring up the next dialog box.

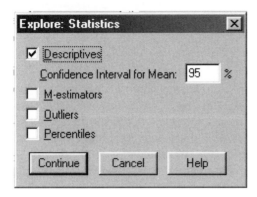

The default option should have the *Descriptives* option selected. Note that you can also select *Percentiles* to generate values corresponding to each percentile. Click *Continue* and then click *OK*. You should then have the following output.

Descriptives

			Statistic	Std. Error
annual household income	Mean		41577.53	587.2969
	95% Confidence Interval for Mean	Lower Bound	40425.84	
		Upper Bound	42729.22	
	5% Trimmed Mean		40069.84	
	Median		36000.00	
	Variance		7.9E + 08	
	Std. Deviation		28061.49	
	Minimum		.00	
	Maximum		110000.0	
	Range		110000.0	
	Interquartile Range		36000.00	
	Skewness		0.716	0.051
	Kurtosis		−0.134	0.102

This output contains both measures of centrality and the dispersion.

We can also compute descriptive statistics using the *Descriptives* option from *Descriptive Statistics* in the *Analyze* menu.

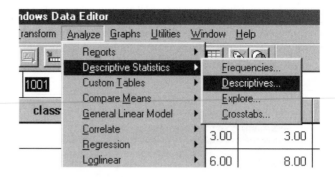

Once the *Descriptives* option has been selected, a dialog box will allow the researcher to select the variable of interest in the usual way. It is possible to control the type of descriptive statistic that is computed by clicking on the *Options* button (located in the lower right-hand corner of the dialog box). Note that the median and interquartile range are not selections in this option. Click on *Continue* and then *OK* to carry out the procedure.

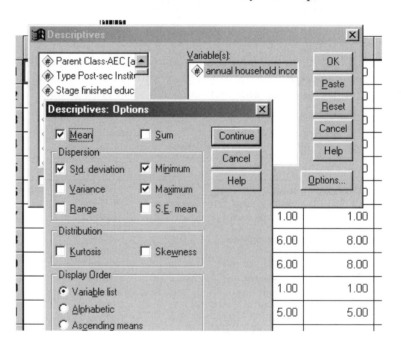

Working with Excel

There are various ways of generating descriptive statistics in Excel. We will confine our discussion to using the *Data Analysis* option in the *Tools* menu.

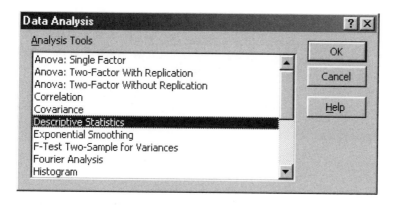

Once we have selected *Data Analysis*, we can select the *Descriptive Statistics* option. The following dialog box will appear.

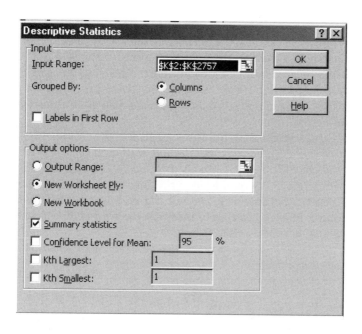

Define in the *Input Range* window the cell range covering the data values you wish to analyse. The values for the variables of interest are in column K. They start in row 2 and end in row 2757. To define these values in the *Input Range* window, you first click on the first data point in column K (this is cell $K$2, that is, the second row in column K). You then type a colon : and click on the cell containing the last data value (this will be cell $K$2757, the 2757th row in column K). Select the option *Summary statistics*, and click *OK*. This procedure should generate the following output in a separate Excel worksheet.

	A	B	(
1	*Column1*		
2			
3	Mean	41577.53	
4	Standard	587.2969	
5	Median	36000	
6	Mode	45000	
7	Standard	28061.49	
8	Sample Va	7.87E+08	
9	Kurtosis	−0.13387	
10	Skewness	0.715966	
11	Range	110000	
12	Minimum	0	
13	Maximum	110000	
14	Sum	94921500	
15	Count	2283	
16			

Both Excel and SPSS can be used to describe data. When new versions of the statistical packages come out there are sometimes changes to the menu tabs and the step-by-step dialog box procedures for deriving those descriptions. However, as long as you are aware of the basic processes for deriving graphical displays, such as summary statistics, you should not have difficulty adapting to any new versions of the software.

Excel is a spreadsheet with built-in statistical and graphing tools. SPSS is a powerful and comprehensive stand-alone statistical package. We saw, for example, that Excel does not readily produce stem and leaf displays or boxplots, although it is possible to write macros to produce these plots. Excel has benefits because it is part of the widely used Microsoft Office suite, making it more accessible to most people with computers.

SUMMARY

Observation does not stop suddenly when the social scientist has defined the variables and collected the statistics. The processes of reasoning about observations – induction, deduction and abduction – continue after the data have been collected. Numbers require analysis and interpretation.

The good statistical sleuth has a number of tools and strategies to assist him or her in the organization and understanding of data. The experienced data snooper explores the data, obtaining summary statistics that give an overview of what is happening. The data snooper can use a table or a figure to highlight important features, including the incongruous, the unexpected and the peculiar. Graphs and figures, however, have limitations – they can be used to exaggerate findings as well as to clarify them. Tabular and visual displays are important in presenting findings and the corresponding arguments, but the good data snooper always asks for the data and checks the validity of the claims being made.

The data from a study normally go into a variable by case matrix – a dataset. The *Accounting for Tastes* project has a relatively large dataset. We can describe the main characteristics of that dataset in terms of its shape, the location or centrality of the data and the dispersion or spread of the data. We discussed a number of summary measures or indices of centrality and dispersion. Measures of centrality provide information about what is typical or average. They are important and useful statistical information. But care needs to be taken when interpreting and discussing measures of centrality. These measures are summary indices and we can lose information on the individual datum – the individual case.

We also considered several measures of variability or dispersion. Measures of centrality provide the statistical sleuth with clues about where most of the data are centred or located. These measures, though, do not provide the sleuth with any information on the variability of the data. A more complete set of clues on a dataset would include an appropriate measure of dispersion. As with measures of centrality, there is no single 'best' measure of variability. The statistical sleuth must choose between dispersion indices and select a measure that is appropriate for the situation.

Understanding the language of statistics – the notation and formulae – is important for making informed decisions about the choice of statistical measures. Each of the measures has a role in understanding the nature of the data and its limitations. We also need to remember that statistical packages are not substitutes for a sound working knowledge of the data analysis procedures. The experienced statistical sleuth will know that certain techniques and measures are appropriate and meaningful for a particular dataset, and then use a spreadsheet or statistical package to carry out the analysis or generate the graphs. Statistical knowledge is indispensable when interpreting output generated by a package. The statistical package will not interpret the output for us – Elementary!

We provide brief lessons on SPSS in the *The Statistical Inquirer* CD-ROM, as well as access to an SPSS data file *computer anxiety.sav* from a study on computer anxiety. Use these lessons and the lessons on descriptive statistics to broaden your knowledge about basic statistical procedures. In Chapter 6, we will continue our exploration of SPSS and Excel as valuable (some would say essential) tools in data analysis.

MAIN POINTS

- Numbers are not neutral. They form patterns and tell a story.
- Good statistical detective work involves making sense of the data collected. We begin our statistical detective work by exploring data.

- Plotting data is a good way of exploring data. There are many ways of representing data visually. Three commonly used methods are stem and leaf displays, boxplots and histograms. We can use these methods to compare distributions and identify salient features of distributions.
- Tables can be used to organize and present information. Tables and graphs should be labelled appropriately and numbered consecutively.
- Large amounts of data can be summarized to account for centrality and variability.
- The mean, mode and median are measures of central tendency or centrality. The median is said to be a resistant statistic because the size of the median is unaffected by extreme values in the distribution.
- The range, standard deviation, variance and interquartile range are measures of dispersion or variability.

REVIEW EXERCISES

1 Statistics students at a regional university complete a confidential survey about each lecturer, indicating to what extent they find the lecturer a likeable person, on a scale from 0 to 7 where 0 means 'not likeable' and 7 means 'very likeable'. Data are collected for 20 lecturers and presented below:

6 3 3 4 3 5 5 6 3 5 2 6 5 5 3 7 5 4 7 2

Construct a stem and leaf display for these data. Comment on the distribution of popularity ratings.

2 Popularity ratings for psychology lecturers are obtained from students at the same regional university as in Question 1. Students rated 20 psychology lecturers on a popularity scale from 0 to 7 where 0 means 'not likeable' and 7 means 'very likeable'. Data are collected for 20 lecturers and presented below:

4 6 7 4 3 6 4 6 3 5 3 6 5 5 4 7 5 6 7 3

Compute the five-number summary and draw a boxplot for these data. Draw a boxplot for the popularity ratings of statistics lecturers and compare this plot with the plot for psychology students. What conclusions can you arrive at by comparing the boxplots for statistics and psychology lecturers?

3 A psychologist examines the effects of environmental noise on mental performance. She randomly selects two groups of students. One group, Group 1, is given a problem-solving task while loud environmental noise is played in the background. The second group, Group 2, completes the same problem-solving task under

quiet conditions. High scores indicate good performance. The scores for the two groups are as follows:

Group 1: 18 20 22 21 15 17 20 26 21
Group 2: 23 23 22 27 22 23 20 20 27

Compute the mean, median and mode for each group. Compare the standard deviations for each group. What can you conclude?

4 Here's an exercise worthy of Sherlock Holmes, famous detective and amateur statistician. Choose any four numbers from 1 to 10; you can repeat a number if you wish. How many ways are there of choosing any four numbers so that the variance of those numbers is as small as possible? How many ways are there of choosing any four numbers so that the variance of those numbers is as large as possible? Does the situation change if repeat numbers are not allowed? (Adapted from Moore and McCabe, 1993: 55.)

5 The sociology department of an Australian university, seeing its staff as solid golfers, decides to enter its staff members in an annual 'Socio-Golf' tournament, an intervarsity tournament. The golf scores of the 15 staff members are:

88 80 85 92 86 88 90 100 103 105 77 76 81 80 75

Compute the standard deviation and interquartile range for these data. Based on the shape of the distribution, what measure of dispersion would you report and why?

6 Derive summary statistics from the dataset *computeranxiety.sav* on *The Statistical Inquirer* CD-ROM. The SPSS lessons on the CD-ROM will give you clues on how to derive summary statistics from the dataset.

REFERENCES

Abelson, R.P. (1995) *Statistics as Principled Argument*. Hillsdale: Lawrence Erlbaum Associates.

Beall, A. (1994) Gender and the perception of evolution. Unpublished doctoral dissertation, Yale University, New Haven, CT.

Bennett, T., Emmison, M. and Frow, J. (1999) *Accounting for Tastes: Australian Everyday Culture*. Cambridge: Cambridge University Press.

Chambers, J.M. et al. (1983) *Graphical Methods for Data Analysis*. Belmont, CA: Duxbury Press.

Christie, A. (1982) *Poirot Loses a Client*. New York: Dell.

Doyle, Arthur Conan (1952) *The Complete Sherlock Holmes*. Garden City, New York: Doubleday.

Farquhar, A.B. and Farquhar, H. (1891) *Economic and Industrial Delusions: A discourse of the case for protection*. New York: Putnam.

Hansel, C.E.M. (1980) *ESP and Parapsychology: A critical re-evaluation*. Buffalo, NY: Prometheus Books.

Ho, R. and Zemaitis, R. (1981) 'Concern over the negative consequences of success', *Australian Journal of Psychology*, 33: 19–28.

Rawstorne, P.R., Caputi, P. and Smith, B. (1998) 'Toward the development of a measure of subjective computer experience'. Unpublished Manuscript, University of Wollongong, Australia.

Rhine, J.B. and Pratt, J.G. (1954) 'A review of the Pearce-Pratt Distance Series of ESP tests', *Journal of Parapsychology*, 18: 165–77.

Sternberg, R.J. (1977) *Writing the Psychology Paper*. Woodbury, NY: Barron's Educational Series.

Tukey, J.W. (1977) *Exploratory Data Analysis*. Reading, MA: Addison-Wesley.

Velleman, P.F. and Hoaglin, D.C. (1981) *Applications, Basics and Computing of Exploratory Data Analysis*. Duxbury Press, Boston.

Wainer, H. (1992) *Understanding Graphs and Tables*. Technical Report No. 92-19. Princeton New Jersey: Educational Testing Service.

6

Finding Answers from the Inquiry

'Elementary, my dear Watson!'

.

Sherlock Holmes had two purposes in mind when he used the word 'elementary'. The first purpose was to demonstrate the brilliance and simplicity of his solution to a problem. The second was to show Dr Watson that the conclusion had to follow from the evidence. Careful collection of evidence and creative insight mark Holmes as the stereotype of the brilliant problem-solver.

The solution to one problem in a crime case, of course, is not necessarily a solution to the whole case. In his cases, Holmes goes through all the stages of research: exploration, collection of data, analysis and findings. The accumulation of clues assists in solving the case, but it is the relationships between those clues that matter most. As the evidence builds up and the detective builds the links between his or her observations, a picture emerges. At a certain point, the detective starts to reconstruct what happened. Ellery Queen, the detective in *The Dutch Shoe Mystery*, reconstructs from his observations what he thought to be the murderer's actions.

10:29 The real Dr Janney called away.

10:30 Lucille Price opens door from Anteroom, slips into Anteroom lift, closes door, fastens East Corridor door to prevent interruptions, dons shoes, white duck trousers, gown, cap and gag previously planted there or somewhere in the Anteroom, leaves her own shoes in elevator, her own clothes being covered by the new. Slips into East Corridor via lift door, turns corner into South Corridor, goes along South Corridor until she reaches Anaesthesia Room. Limping all the time, in imitation of Janney, with gag concealing her features and cap her hair, she passes rapidly through the Anaesthesia Room, being seen by Dr Byers, Miss Obermann and Cudahy, and enters Anteroom, closing door behind her.

10:34 Approaches comatose Mrs. Doorn, strangles her with wire concealed under her clothes; calls out in her own voice at appropriate time, 'I'll be out in a moment, Dr Janney!' or words to that effect. (Of course, she did not go into the Sterilizing Room as she claimed in her testimony.) When Dr Gold stuck his head into the Anteroom he saw Miss Price in surgical robes bending over the body, her back to him. Naturally Gold did not see a nurse; there was none, as such, there.

10:38 Leaves Anteroom through Anaethesia Room, retraces steps along South and East Corridors, slips into lift, removes male garments, puts on own shoes, hurries out again to deposit male clothes in telephone booth just outside lift door, and returns to Anteroom via lift door as before.

10:43 Is back in Anteroom in her own personality as Lucille Price. (Queen, 1983: 234–5)

'The entire process consumed no more than twelve minutes', says Queen.

Ellery Queen is right. Lucille Price killed Mrs Doorn, the hospital's benefactor. But there is more to the story. Why did Price kill Doorn? And was anyone else involved? Each step in the problem-solving process leads to other steps. The detective has to decide not only which observations count as clues, but also which relationships between clues are useful and meaningful. We have already raised some of these issues in the discussion on validity in Chapter 4.

The social scientist can learn from the idea of the detective as the data collector and creative problem-solver, as Innes (1965) points out in his critique of Sherlock Holmes. 'Before any solution can appear the subject must perceive that a problem exists' (1965: 12). Holmes, like Ellery Queen, is sensitive to deficiencies in evidence and he is able to identify 'gaps' in the evidence. Holmes is motivated by curiosity in the unique and novel, 'the incongruous' (1965: 14). This ability relies on more than 'rational' and 'deductive' processes. It also relies on emotive and evaluative processes that associate previously unrelated ideas. The creative genius Isaac Newton, Innes notes, also engaged in detective work (1965: 15).

Linking ideas together is a creative act, but empirical evidence – observations – assist in this process. Holmes was systematic in his collection and recording of information for future reference. He had a card index of criminals and news items.

> At all times he practises his ability to notice fine details and to make judgements as to the character of his client and of the criminal on the basis of his previous knowledge. An example will make this clearer. In the tale of the *Red-Headed League* Holmes makes the following observation.
>
>> 'Beyond the obvious facts that he has at some time done manual labour, that he takes snuff, that he is a Freemason, that he has been in China, and that he has done a considerable amount of writing lately, I can deduce nothing else.'
>
> After being asked the obvious question by his prompt, Dr Watson, Holmes goes on to observe that the man's right hand is a size larger than his left, that he wears a breast pin of an arc and compass, that his right sleeve is very shiny for five inches and the left has a smooth patch where it has rested on the desk, and finally that on his right wrist he has a tattoo mark stained in a manner only practised in China. This last point is important, as Holmes is able to make this comment because he has contributed to the literature on tattoo marks. Had it not been for this expert knowledge then he could have made no such deduction. (Innes, 1965: 12–13)

The process of collecting data and creating theories can occur at the same time. Some insights about data can only be made if the detective has prior knowledge. In detective fiction, though, there is an end point – the solution – to a series of problems. There is a point in the detective narrative at which a decision is made on how the observations and the relationships between clues solve the case.

In this chapter we go a step beyond exploration of data. In quantitative studies we often wish to explore the relationships between variables and to fit those relationships to theories. We will investigate both the statistical side and the theoretical side of this process.

LOOKING AT BIVARIATE DATA, CORRELATION AND REGRESSION

In the previous chapter we examined ways of exploring, describing and summarizing data from a single variable – *univariate* analysis of data. We examined a range of graphical and numerical methods for representing univariate data. But most variables do not exist in isolation. Social scientists are often interested in the relationships between two or more variables. A clinical psychologist may be interested in the relationship between depression and a schizophrenic's belief in hearing voices. This would be an example of a bivariate analysis – a study of the relationship between two variables. The clinical psychologist may also be interested in the relationship between more than two variables. We would then be involved in analysis of *multivariate* relationships.

It is beyond the compass of this book to cover the statistical techniques for multivariate analysis, but we will explore the statistical techniques for analysing bivariate relationships. We will continue our investigation into the role of graphical and numerical methods for describing variables and the strength, relationship and direction of variables.

Plotting Bivariate Data

We can represent bivariate data (pairs of data values) graphically on a two-dimensional plot known as a scatterplot. Scatterplots are also known as scatter diagrams. The basic idea of a scatterplot is that each pair of data values can be represented as a point on a two-dimensional plot. For example, consider the hypothetical data in Table 6.1 for two variables X and Y.

TABLE 6.1   Hypothetical data

Person	X	Y
1	9	7
2	12	8
3	5	4
4	6	7
5	2	4
6	4	3

We can represent the data for person 2 as the set of coordinates (12, 8). The number '12' means that the X value is 12 units along the measurement represented by the X-axis; the number '8' signifies that the Y value is 8 units along the Y-axis. The scale values for the X and Y-axes begin with 0. The scatterplot in Figure 6.1 displays the bivariate Table 6.1 data.

Figure 6.1 shows that as the values of X increase, the values of Y increase and vice versa. There is a *positive relationship* between X and Y. The statistical sleuth might also find that a scatterplot for X and Y may show that X and Y have a negative relationship. High values on one variable are associated with low values on the second variable, as in Figure 6.2

On the other hand, it may be difficult to see any systematic relationship between X and Y, indicating that the two variables are *not related* (Figure 6.3).

Scatterplots may also form a strong cluster, as though around a line, indicating that the relationship between X and Y is *linear*. It is also possible that the scatter forms a curve, indicating a non-linear relationship between X and Y.

As we found in the last chapter, graphical techniques can also be useful in identifying *outliers* or values that are very different from the general trend

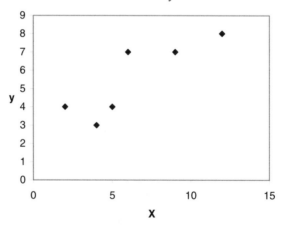

FIGURE 6.1   *Scatterplot for data in Table 6.1*

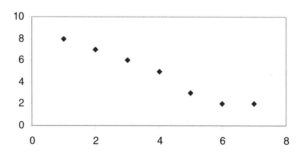

FIGURE 6.2   *Negative association between two variables*

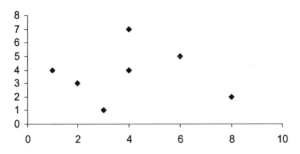

FIGURE 6.3   *No relationship between two variables*

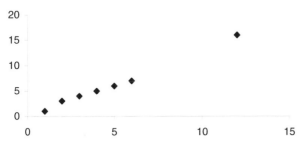

FIGURE 6.4   *Scatterplot showing an outlier*

represented by the rest of the data. A scatterplot can also be used to identify outliers, as you can see in Figure 6.4.

What should the data snooper do when there is evidence of outliers in the data? The first step should always be to check the data for data entry errors. There is nothing more frustrating than conducting a series of analyses, agonizing over the interpretation of results that were unexpected, only to find that the results are influenced by a data entry error. Check for mistakes in recording the data. If you eliminate data entry error as an explanation for the outlier, you should then check that the data themselves are valid, that is, that the data points are faithful and accurate representations of the variables being measured. If the data are valid then a detailed examination of the outliers (and any other characteristics of the individuals whose data are different) may lead to revision of the theoretical underpinning of the study.

The data snooper may also find that the points on a scatterplot cluster into groups. This type of pattern may suggest that there are distinct groups of individuals that should be analysed separately. Alternatively, it may suggest the need for a third dimension (in other words another variable!) to explain why the data are clustering.

Correlation: a Measure of Co-Relation

With scatterplots we pair one observation with another observation. From a scatterplot we can identify trends and patterns among a collection of paired observations. Scatterplots are a useful visual aid but it is also possible to create a simple summary description (a numerical summary) of the degree of relationship. This is the role of correlation.

Like the scatterplot, correlation is a relation – a relation between paired observations. Correlation is also concerned with covariation – how two variables covary. A psychologist may be interested in how delinquency and parental bonding covary. If there is evidence of correlation and co-variation between delinquency and parental bonding, our psychologist may wonder whether delinquency can be estimated from parental bonding. While *correlation* is concerned with the degree and direction of relation between two variables, *prediction* is concerned with estimation, that is, estimating one variable from another variable.

Historically, the concept of prediction precedes any mathematical or stat-istical development of correlation. In 1885, Sir Francis Galton, a gentleman scholar, published an influential paper titled 'Regression towards medioc-rity in hereditary stature' – a paper that also had implications for the the-ories of evolution for Galton's cousin, Sir Charles Darwin. Galton used *regression* to refer to certain observations that he had made. He noticed that tall parents did not always have tall offspring. In fact, on average, the children of tall parents tended to be shorter than their parents; and short parents tended, on average, to have taller offspring. Statisticians now refer to this phenomenon as regression towards the mean. The term regression no longer has the biological connotation. But Galton's ideas on regression were developed by Sir Karl Pearson and resulted in a measure of co-relation, namely the correlation coefficient. In fact, the most widely used measure of correlation is known as the *Pearson Product Moment Correlation*.

We saw that certain features of bivariate data can be identified from a scatterplot. We can see by eye whether two variables are positively or negatively related, or if they are related at all. We can also establish whether the relationship is linear. The correlation coefficient or simply correlation is a numerical summary depicting the strength or magnitude of the relationship that we see by eye, as well as a measure of the direction of the relationship.

Variables like height can be measured in centimetres or inches. But in measuring bivariate relationships we want to be confident that we can measure the strength of the relationship between variables irrespective of whether height is measured in centimetres or inches, or whether age is measured in years or months, and so on. One way of removing the influ-ence of scaling is to standardize the variables. To standardize a variable we simply subtract from the variable score the mean of that variable and divide by the standard deviation of that variable. If X is a variable with mean M and standard deviation s, the standardized version of X, which we will denote as Z_X, is

$$Z_X = \frac{X - M}{s}$$

If John's exam score is 4, the mean of the exam scores is 5.75 and the standard deviation is 2.11, then the standardized score would be -0.83. John's score is, therefore, 0.83 standard deviations below the mean. The Pearson Product Moment Correlation Coefficient or simply, Pearson's correlation coefficient, is a numerical summary of a bivariate relationship. It is defined in terms of standardized variables. Let Z_X and Z_Y denote the standardized variables for X and Y respectively. Pearson's correlation coefficient, r, is defined as

$$r = \frac{\sum Z_X Z_Y}{n - 1}$$

where n is the number of pairs of observations. This measure is the average product of the standardized variables. The coefficient, r, is obtained by standardizing each variable, summing their product and dividing by $n - 1$. Some statistics texts will define r as

$$r = \frac{\sum Z_X Z_Y}{n}.$$

That is, n rather than $n - 1$ will divide the sum of the product of standardized variables. The latter formula is used if you are analysing a population. The former equation is used if you are analysing a sample. We will return to the distinction between samples and populations.

The process of standardizing scores was important in the development of the correlation coefficient. Like the good, modern-day data snooper, Galton began by producing a scatterplot of the parents and their respective offspring. Galton's scatterplot was perhaps the first of its kind. He standardized all heights. He then computed the means of the children's standardized heights and compared them to fixed values of the standardized heights of corresponding parents.

What Galton found was that the means tended to fall along a straight line. What was more remarkable was that the each mean height of the children deviated less from their overall mean height than the parents deviated from their overall mean. There was a tendency for the mean height of the offspring to move toward the overall mean. This observation was in fact an instance of a correlation that is not perfect. In fact, the correlation was about 0.5 (Guilford, 1965).

There are many ways of re-expressing the formula for r. All of these alternative formulae are equivalent. An alternative formula that is easier computationally is

$$r = \frac{n \sum XY - \left(\sum X \right)\left(\sum Y \right)}{n(n - 1)s_X s_Y}$$

Having said that this equation is easier computationally, it is usual practice to use a calculator, statistical package or spreadsheet program to compute r rather than compute the coefficient by hand.

Example 6.1: Computing the correlation coefficient

Do sports psychologists become more effective as they become more experienced? A university researcher studied a random sample of 10 psychologists, each of whom was seeing athletes with similar problems. The researcher measured the number of sessions needed for a noticeable improvement in athletes as well as the number of years of experience for each sports psychologist. The data are presented in Table 6.2. Is there a correlation between years of experience and effective outcome?

TABLE 6.2   *Hypothetical data on correlation between years of counselling experience and effective outcome*

Years of experience	No. of sessions
5	9
8	7
8	9
7	6
6	10
4	12
2	10
9	7
10	6
8	7

To find the correlation we use the formula:

$$r = \frac{n\sum XY - \left(\sum X\right)\left(\sum Y\right)}{n(n-1)s_X s_Y}$$

Let years of experience be the variable X and number of sessions the variable Y. We compute the standard deviations of X and Y and find that $S_X = 2.45$ and $S_Y = 2.00$. We also find that $\sum X = 67$ and $\sum Y = 83$ and $\sum XY = 522$. There are 10 sports psychologists, $n = 10$. Substituting these values into the correlation equation we have:

$$r = \frac{10(522) - (67)(83)}{10(10-1)(2.45)(2.00)}$$

$$r = \frac{-341}{441}$$

$$r = -0.773$$

The correlation between years of experience and number of sessions is −0.773. There is a strong negative correlation between these variables which indicates that more experienced psychologists arrive at effective outcomes with clients in fewer sessions than inexperienced psychologists.

The correlation coefficient has some important properties. The magnitude of the correlation coefficient indicates the strength of the relationship between the variables. The values of the correlation coefficient can range from −1 to +1. A coefficient close to +1 or −1 indicates a strong relationship between two variables. Values close to zero indicate the absence of a relationship between two variables. If the coefficient has a negative sign, then the variables are negatively associated. If the coefficient has a positive sign, then the variables are positively related.

Perhaps most importantly, and a fact that is sometimes overlooked by inexperienced statistical sleuths, is that the correlation coefficient is a measure of linear association. In other words, if we were to fit a straight line through the swarm of points on a scatterplot representing a perfect linear association, all the points would lie on the line.

If the relationship is curvilinear, the correlation coefficient can be misleading. Consider the scatterplot in Figure 6.5 for two variables X and Y.

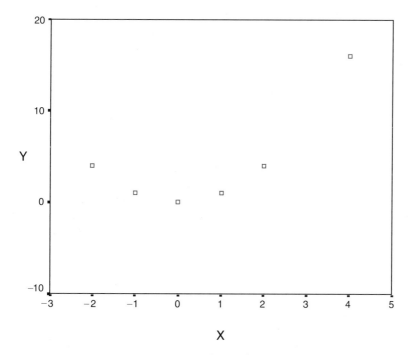

FIGURE 6.5   A curvilinear relationship

TABLE 6.3   *Data with outliers*

Person	X	Y
1	1	5
2	4	3
3	5	2
4	4	5
5	5	8
6	6	7
7	12	14

The plot suggests that the relationship between X and Y is not linear. However, the correlation coefficient for these data is 0.73, suggesting a strong linear association. But clearly the relationship is curvilinear, not linear. This shows the importance of plotting your data as one way of checking that the underlying assumptions of a particular statistical procedure or measure are met. It also shows the importance of not relying on just one piece of evidence to make decisions!

In Chapter 5 we introduced the concept of resistant statistics. You will recall that a resistant statistic is unaffected by extreme values. The correlation coefficient is not a resistant statistic. Consider the hypothetical data for two variables X and Y collected from seven people, shown in Table 6.3.

If we consider the data for the first six people we find that the correlation between X and Y is 0.20. The data for seventh person represents a possible outlier. If we include the data for the seventh person, the correlation coefficient is $r = 0.80$. The inclusion of the outlier yields a strong correlation, but when the outlier is omitted the correlation between X and Y is quite weak. This example further highlights the importance of plotting data.

Introduction to Simple Linear Regression

Quite often social scientists are interested in predicting one variable based on information from another variable. A psychologist, for instance, may be interested in predicting coffee or tea consumption from work stress. In the case of prediction, we then use the language of *explanatory variable* (work stress) and *response variable* (coffee or tea consumption). The psychologist may wish to go beyond simply saying that stress and caffeine consumption are associated. There is a technique that allows us to describe the relationship between explanatory and response variables in a linear form. This procedure is known as *simple linear regression*.

Prediction and Correlation

Prediction and correlation are closely related concepts. If two variables X and Y are unrelated, then knowing something about X tells us nothing about Y. It is not possible to accurately predict Y from X in this situation. In fact guessing would be as good a prediction as we could get! However, if X and Y are related, then knowing something about X implies some knowledge of Y. In this case, we can go beyond a simple guess and predict Y from X with some accuracy. As the correlation between X and Y increases, the accuracy with which we can predict Y from X also increases (Ferguson, 1959).

We need to be careful, however, about the meaning of the term 'prediction'. For the layperson, prediction implies being able to determine something exactly. In other words, it implies causation. Statistically, prediction is closely related to *estimation*. Although we say that X predicts Y we must remember that prediction is still based on correlation. We can predict something but only with a certain level of accuracy and confidence. We will return to these and related issues later.

Method of Least Squares

We have used scatterplots to investigate not just the presence of a relationship between two variables X and Y but also whether that relationship is linear. If there is evidence of linearity, then the straight line is the simplest way of describing Y from X. That is, we can *model* Y from X. The most commonly used approach of modelling or fitting a line to bivariate data is the *method of least squares*.

The method of least squares seeks to find a line of best fit through the swarm of points on a scatterplot. But how do we define 'best fit'? If we wish to describe a line predicting Y from X then we position the line through the points such that we minimize the sum of the squared distances taken parallel to the Y axis from each point to the line. The idea is illustrated in Figure 6.6.

The line passing through the points represents the predicted responses. We use the symbolic language $\hat{y}$ to denote these predicted responses. The distance between a point and the line represents the difference between predicted and observed y values, $y - \hat{y}$. These differences are also referred to as the *residuals* and are illustrated in Figure 6.7.

The method of least squares aims to fit a line so that the sum of the squared residuals is minimized. In other words, if the line is a good

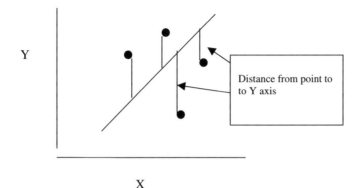

Y

Distance from point to
to Y axis

X

FIGURE 6.6   *Fitting a line through points on a scatterplot*

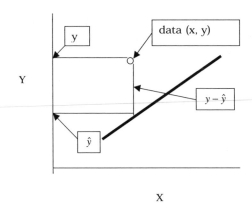

FIGURE 6.7   *Illustrating the concept of residual*

model (that is, good prediction) the residual values will be as small as possible. The smaller the residuals the better the fit of the line to the data. The general equation for a straight line is

$$y = a + bx$$

where a is the intercept and b is the slope of the line. The intercept is the distance on the Y-axis from the origin to where the line cuts the Y-axis. In other words, it is the value of Y when $X = 0$. The slope of the line is an indication of the rate of change of Y as X changes. That is, the rate of increase in Y as X increases. It is beyond the scope of this introductory book to present the mathematical derivation of the estimates of a and b when the least squares method is applied. Suffice it to say that we can calculate the values of a and b using the following equations:

$$b = \frac{\sum xy - \frac{1}{n}\left(\sum x\right)\left(\sum y\right)}{\sum x^2 - \frac{1}{n}\left(\sum x\right)^2}$$

$$a = M_y - bM_x$$

where M_y and M_x are the means of the Y and X values respectively. Statistical texts also represent the means of Y and X symbolically as $\bar{y}$ and $\bar{x}$ respectively.

Once we have estimated the values of a and b, we are in a position to predict values of Y, $\hat{y}$. We can use the following equation, also known as a *regression equation*, to predict $\hat{y}$:

$$\hat{y} = a + bx$$

Let's return for a moment to our psychologist who is interested in predicting caffeine consumption from the amount of work stress. In this case, x would represent known values of work stress. Stress might be measured using an *inventory*, a test or set of tests, that yields scores between 0 and 20 where low scores indicate minimal stress and high scores high levels of stress. Caffeine consumption is measured in terms of the number of cups of tea or coffee consumed per day.

Let's now assume that the regression from predicting caffeine consumption from stress scores is given by the regression equation, $\hat{y} = 3 + 0.7x$. We interpret the slope of the line 0.7 to mean that there is a caffeine consumption increase by 0.7 of a cup for every unit increase in the stress score. The intercept, which has a value of 3, would be the caffeine consumption if a person had a score of 0. We can also use this equation to predict values of caffeine consumption from any value of work stress. For example, if a person scores 12 on the work stress inventory, we can predict (on the basis of the regression equation) that he or she consumes $11.4[3 + 0.7(12)]$ cups of coffee or tea per day.

Example 6.2: Finding the regression line

Let us return to the data in Table 6.2 and find the regression predicting the number of sessions required for effective outcome in terms of years of experience. To find the regression line we need to compute the constant a and the slope b. Using the following equations:

$$b = \frac{\sum xy - \frac{1}{n}\left(\sum x\right)\left(\sum y\right)}{\sum x^2 - \frac{1}{n}\left(\sum x\right)^2} \quad \text{and} \quad a = M_y - bM_x$$

We find that $\sum XY = 522$, $\sum X = 67$, $\sum Y = 83$, $\sum X^2 = 503$ and $\left(\sum X\right)^2 = 4489$.

Substituting these values into the formula for b we have:

$$b = \frac{\sum xy - \frac{1}{n}\left(\sum x\right)\left(\sum y\right)}{\sum x^2 - \frac{1}{n}\left(\sum x\right)^2}$$

$$b = \frac{522 - (67)(83)/10}{503 - (4489)/10}$$

$$b = \frac{-34.1}{54.1}$$

$$b = -0.63$$

$$a = M_y - bM_x$$

$$a = 8.3 - (-0.63)(6.7)$$

$$a = 12.52$$

Therefore our regression equation is $\hat{y} = 12.52 - 0.63x$.

The Statistical Inquirer multimedia courseware covers correlation and regression. Use the exercises in the course to further develop your skill in using the statistic. Remember to use the dataset to assist the practice.

Assessing the Fit of the Regression Model

There are a number of ways of assessing how well our regression equation, the model for predicting the response variable from the explanatory variable, fits the data. We have already said that good prediction requires the residuals to be as small as possible. If the regression model is adequate then the predicted values based on the regression model will be close to the actual values. In other words, when the statistical sleuth has an acceptable regression model for bivariate data, the residuals will all be close to zero. Having lots of large residuals is an indication that the model is not fitting the data well. There may be instances where the model does not fit one or two of the values. This is evidence that those values are potential outliers.

Residuals can be thought of as the error one makes in estimating the values of a response variable – they are errors of estimation. The standard deviation of these errors is a handy measure of the accuracy of the estimate. It is a measure of the accuracy of predicting the response variable Y from knowing something about the explanatory variable X. This measure is also known as the *standard error of the estimate*, $s_{y \cdot x}$, and is given the equation:

$$s_{y \cdot x} = \sqrt{\frac{\sum (y - \hat{y})^2}{n}}$$

The values for a response variable Y consist of two parts, a component that is estimated, $\hat{y}$, and a component corresponding to the error of estimation, $y - \hat{y}$. If we think of the estimated value as the model for Y, and the error of estimation as the residual, then any data point can be defined in terms of a model component and a residual component.

$$\text{Data} = \text{model} + \text{residual}$$

The variances of the model and residual components are additive. Moreover, the variance of a response variable is equal to the sum of the variance of the model and residual components. In other words, the variance of Y, s_y^2, is equal to the sum of the variance of the predicted value of Y, $s_{\hat{y}}^2$, and the variance of the residuals, $s_{y \cdot x}^2$. The ratio of the variance of the predicted values of Y and the variance of the observed values of Y has a special relationship with the correlation coefficient. The ratio of these variances is equal to the square of the correlation coefficient:

$$r^2 = \frac{s_{\hat{y}}^2}{s_y^2}$$

This ratio shows the amount of variance of the response variable that is explained by the regression model. This ratio is also known as the *coefficient of determination*. It provides one way of assessing the adequacy of the regression model. If r^2 is 0.70 we can state that 70 per cent of the variance in Y is explained by the regression model. This result suggests that the regression model is accounting for a considerable amount of the variance in the response variable. In some texts the coefficient of determination is represented symbolically as R^2.

A final caveat! It is important that the data snooper considers all the evidence available when making a decision about the adequacy of a regression line or model. Begin by looking at a scatterplot of the data to see if the relationship is linear. Then examine the measures we have just discussed to determine the 'goodness' of fit of the regression line. More advanced and detailed treatments of the topic of regression are available in texts by Draper and Smith (1981), Kerlinger and Pedhazur (1973) and Cohen and Cohen (1983).

Issue of Causation

We know that there is a correlation between smoking and lung cancer. There is supporting evidence that heavy smokers tend to contract lung cancer more frequently than do non-smokers (US Surgeon General, 1964). But does smoking *cause* lung cancer? Most of the evidence is based on correlational studies comparing cancer rates across different groups. Is the existence of a correlation indicative of a causal relationship?

A correlation between two variables indicates a functional relationship. The values of the response variable appear to be a function of the explanatory variable. But a correlation does not necessarily imply a causal relationship between two variables. Indeed, it is usual for causal conclusions from correlations to be met with severe criticism from the research community. One reason for this criticism is the influence a third variable may have on the correlation between variables X and Y. The claim that smoking causes lung cancer, based on strong correlational evidence, is challenged by critics who assert among other things that smokers on average are more stressed and tense than non-smokers. Therefore we cannot rule out that it is stress or tension that makes smokers vulnerable to lung cancer. In other words, the correlation between smoking and cancer may be due to the influence of a third variable, namely, stress.

There are a number of possible explanations as to why two variables, X and Y, may be strongly associated (Moore and McCabe, 1993). The first explanation is that X causes Y or Y causes X. Here the researcher would need to establish that a change in one variable produces or causes a change in the second. If smoking causes lung cancer then increased smoking will result in lung cancer. The second type of explanation involves the presence of a third factor, Z, influencing the relationship between X and Y. X and Y may be related because X and Y respond to a third variable Z. In this case, we may well be able to, say, predict Y from X, but there are instances where changes to X will not necessarily result in a change in Y. Some researchers have hypothesized that some people are genetically predisposed to certain smoking behaviours and lung cancer. If a person is genetically predisposed to cancer then changes to smoking behaviour will not change the likelihood of contracting cancer.

Another possible explanation for a relationship between two variables is that the effect of one variable on the second is confounded by the influence of a third variable. It may be the case that smokers are more stressed than the average person and therefore, the person is more vulnerable to cancer. It may be that a person who smokes is less careful about their general health and again may be more vulnerable to cancer than someone who is more health conscious. In other words, it is difficult to see which variable is actually associated with cancer. Smoking may be influential, but it would be difficult to discern a causal link between smoking and cancer without removing the influence of the confounding variable.

That said: don't smoke! In the case of research on smoking, there has also been a build-up of various types of evidence, experimental, survey, and so on, over time, that provides support for the causal hypothesis. We have presented a simplistic interpretation of correlations linking smoking and lung cancer. The situation is more complicated than has been presented in this brief discussion. In general, causal statements based on single correlations are fraught with danger. However, if there is evidence of patterns of correlations linking two variables across different groups, then the possibility of a casual link increases. Statistical techniques such as regression, particularly multiple regression, are useful in controlling for third variable influences. In particular, the family of techniques known as structural equation modelling (SEM) allows the researcher to test and confirm models of relationships between sets of variables, thus providing reasonable rejoinders to critics proposing the influence of other variables. By using these techniques we are able to statistically control and test the impact of other variables. Although SEM techniques have grown in popularity, some theorists have reservations on the indiscriminate or inappropriate use of the technique. We are again reminded that a sound understanding of statistical knowledge is essential for both interpretation and use of statistical procedures.

USING SPSS: CORRELATION AND REGRESSION

To illustrate how SPSS provides correlation and regression, we will use Patrick Rawstorne's dataset Predicting and Explaining the use of Information Technology with Value Expectancy Models of Behaviour in Contexts of Mandatory Use. This is the dataset provided in *The Statistical Inquirer* for your practice.

The dataset examines the relationship between personality measures, computer anxiety and subjective computer experience. One research question of interest in this study is whether there is a relationship between neuroticism and computer anxiety. To examine this question, we begin by generating a scatterplot for neuroticism and computer anxiety. The two variables are labelled 'neurotic' and 'anxiety1' respectively. We can generate a scatterplot in SPSS by going to the *Graphs* menu and selecting *Scatter*.

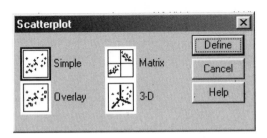

Once you select *Scatter*, you will get the following dialog box.

Click on *Simple* and then choose *Define*. The next dialog box will ask you to select the variables you wish to plot.

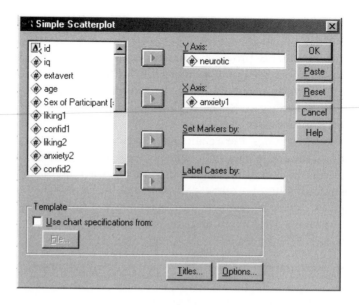

We wish to plot the variables 'neurotic' and 'anxiety1'. We select 'neurotic' and move it to the Y-axis box, and select 'anxiety1' and move it to the X-axis box. Click *OK*. These steps should generate the following output:

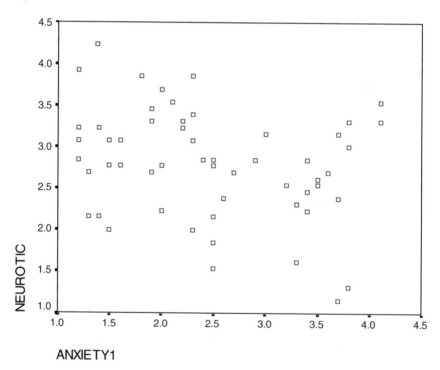

This scatterplot suggests weak negative relationship between the two variables. There is a tendency (weak though it may be) in these data for less neurotic subjects to be more computer anxious. The correlation coefficient will provide a numerical summary of this relationship.

We can obtain a numerical summary of this relationship by computing the correlation coefficient. To do this we select *Correlate* from the *Analyze* menu and then choose *Bivariate*.

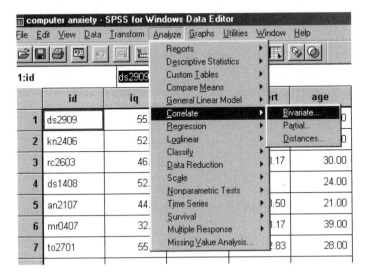

This option allows the user to run Pearson's correlation.

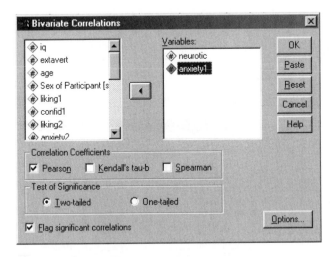

From the *Bivariate Correlations* dialog box, you select the variables 'neurotic' and 'anxiety1' and move them to the *Variables* window. Click on *OK* to run the procedure and obtain the following output.

Correlations

		NEUROTIC	ANXIETY1
NEUROTIC	Pearson Correlation	1.000	−0.276*
	Sig. (2-tailed)		0.038
	N	57	57
ANXIETY1	Pearson Correlation	−0.276*	1.000
	Sig. (2-tailed)	0.038	
	N	57	60

*Correlation is significant at the 0.05 level (2-tailed)

The correlation coefficient is −0.276, a weak negative correlation. The output also gives the p-value associated with the correlation, $p = 0.038$. This value provides support for rejection of a null hypothesis that the population parameter is equal to zero. The 'null hypothesis' is the hypothesis of 'no difference'. The 'p value' is the estimate that the differences claimed by the hypothesis are significant. The convention is to set the significance figure at less than 0.05 or 0.01. We will return to the problem of hypothesis testing and significance in the section on samples and populations.

Can we express the relationship between 'neurotic' and 'anxiety1' as a straight line? Of course, this is done using regression analysis. To conduct a regression analysis in SPSS, select *Regression* from the *Analyze* menu and then choose *Linear*.

This selection will open the *Linear Regression* dialog box.

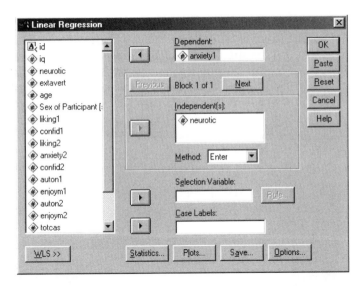

We choose 'neurotic' and move it to the *Independent(s)* window. This is the explanatory variable. The variable 'anxiety1' is the response variable or dependent variable – we move this variable to the *Dependent* window. Click on *OK* to run the procedure. Below is some selected output from the regression analysis.

Model Summary

Model	R	R Square	Adjusted R Square	Std. Error of the Estimate
1	0.276[a]	0.076	0.059	0.8512

[a] Predictors: (Constant), NEUROTIC

This first output shows R^2 and the standard error of the estimate. R^2 is 0.076, indicating that only 7.6 per cent of the variance in 'anxiety1' is explained by 'neurotic'. This value is low, suggesting that the fit of the line to the data is not as good as it could be.

Coefficients[a]

Model		Unstandardized Coefficients		Standardized Coefficients		
		B	Std. Error	Beta	t	Sig.
1	(Constant)	3.513	0.503		6.988	0.000
	NEUROTIC	-0.374	0.176	-0.276	-2.126	0.038

[a] Dependent Variable: ANXIETY 1

This output window contains the values for the slope and intercept of the regression line. The slope is also referred to as a regression coefficient. The intercept is referred to as the constant. There are two types of regression coefficient reported in this output, unstandardized and standardized. The standardized coefficient is based on the standardized values of 'neurotic' and 'anxiety1'. We will use the unstandardized coefficients to construct the equation. The equation is $\hat{y} = 3.513 - 0.374x$ where $\hat{y} =$ 'anxiety1' and $x =$ 'neurotic'.

Using Excel

We can construct a scatterplot in Excel by highlighting the variables you wish to analyse by clicking on the column that defines the variable.

	C	D	E	F	G	H	
IQ	NEUROTIC	EXTAVERT	AGE	SEX	LIKING1	ANXIETY1	COM
.00	4.23	3.33	44.00	2.00	3.50	1.38	
.00	1.15	1.83	43.00	2.00	2.89	3.70	
.00	3.54	3.17	30.00	2.00	2.22	4.10	
.00	#NULL!	#NULL!	24.00	2.00	3.67	1.10	
.00	3.15	3.50	21.00	2.00	2.33	3.70	
.00	2.85	3.17	39.00	2.00	3.56	2.40	
.00	2.69	2.83	28.00	2.00	3.44	2.70	
.00	3.69	3.08	36.00	2.00	3.25	2.00	
.00	2.38	3.33	30.00	2.00	3.78	2.60	

A scatterplot can be constructed by choosing the chart wizard and clicking on XY(*Scatter*). Simply click on *Next* until you reach the end of the step, then click *Finish*.

Your output should now look as follows:

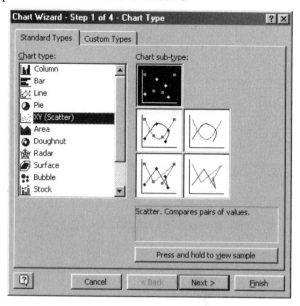

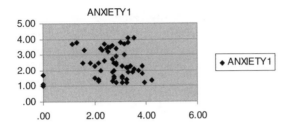

In order to use Excel to carry out a correlation analysis you will need to ensure that the variables are in adjacent columns and that there are no pairs of data with missing values. If you have missing values, as we have with the computer anxiety data, then you should omit those pairs from the analysis by deleting them. Once you have organized the data, you use the data analysis tool package available in Excel to compute the correlation. You select *Data Analysis* from the *Tools* menu.

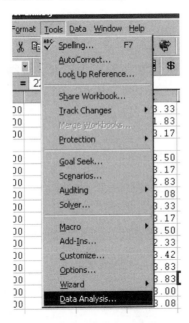

From the *Data Analysis* dialog box select *Correlation*.

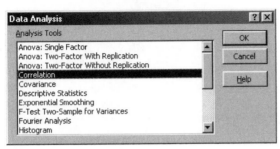

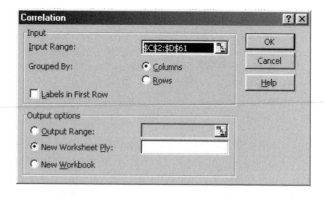

You will need to define the range of cells containing the data in the *Input Range* window. This can be done by highlighting the data to be analysed. Click on OK to compute the correlation.

A regression analysis is also relatively straightforward in Excel. From the *Tools* menu select *Data Analysis*. From the *Data Analysis* dialog box choose *Regression*.

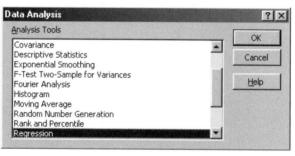

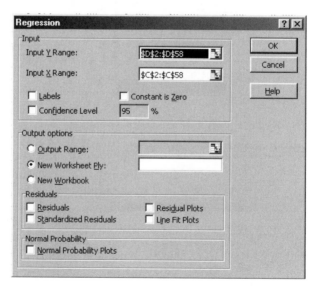

In the *Regression* dialog box you need to define the cell range for the response variable 'anxiety1'. This variable is located in column D and the data is in row 2 through to row 58, the range is $C2:$C58. This cell range is placed in the *Input Y Range* window. The cell range for the explanatory variable 'neurotic' is placed in the *Input X Range* window. Click on *OK* to run the simple linear regression. A snapshot of the output from the Excel regression analysis is presented below.

SUMMARY OUTPUT					
Regression Statistics					
Multiple R	0.275562208				
R Square	0.075934531				
Adjusted R Square	0.05913334				
Standard Error	0.85124823				
Observations	57				
ANOVA					
	df	*SS*	*MS*	*F*	*Si*
Regression	1	3.275003022	3.275003022	4.519592309	
Residual	55	39.85429522	0.72462355		
Total	56	43.12929825			
	Coefficients	*Standard Error*	*t Stat*	*P-value*	
Intercept	3.512979115	0.502704245	6.988162827	3.94432E−09	
X Variable 1	−0.3735443	0.175708384	−2.12593328	0.038013135	

LOOKING AT CATEGORICAL DATA

An important assumption underlying the correlation coefficient is that the variables need to be continuous. There exist, however, a family of techniques for examining the relationship between categorical variables. Many studies in sociology and media studies involve the use of categorical data. Before discussing these techniques we will consider some graphical and tabular methods for exploring bivariate categorical variables.

EXPLORING BIVARIATE CATEGORICAL DATA

Table 6.4 describes the results of the 1836 Pinckney Gag rule, a rule of historical importance because of its role in the antislavery petitions in the US. US congressmen were classified according to the section of the country they represented. These data are from Benson and Oslick (1969), reported in Bishop et al. (1975: 99).

There are two categorical variables represented in Table 6.4, Vote and Section. Vote has three categories or levels, yea, abstain and nay; the

TABLE 6.4   *Distribution of votes by section*

| Section | Distribution of votes | | | |
	Yes	Abstain	No	Total
North	61	12	60	133
Border	17	6	1	24
South	39	22	7	68
Total	117	40	68	225

Source: Bishop et al., 1975

TABLE 6.5   *Percentage of votes within each section*

Section	Yes	Abstain	No
North	46	9	45
Border	71	25	4
South	57	32	10

Source: Bishop et al., 1975

variable Section also has three categories, North, Border and South. These data can be represented graphically as a bar chart in Figure 6.8.

The vertical axis represents the frequency of responses. The horizontal axis represents the three categories for Vote. Within each category of Section, the three categories of the variable Vote are represented. The chart is an effective way of displaying the frequency of voting pattern within sections. However, a comparison of voting with each section is not easy. If the voting data within each section are expressed as a percentage, then a comparison is straightforward. Table 6.5 presents the frequencies within each section expressed as a percentage.

A bar chart using the percentages in Table 6.5 is presented in Figure 6.9. We note that fewer congressmen from the North voted for the rule, quite a different interpretation from the bar chart for Table 6.4. A reading of the raw frequencies shows that Northerners appeared to have more votes but clearly there are more Northern congressmen. Interpreting the raw frequencies is quite misleading!

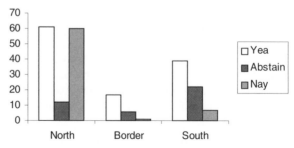

FIGURE 6.8   *Bar chart of frequency of votes by selection*

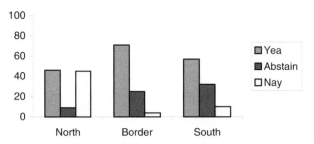

FIGURE 6.9   *Bar chart of raw percentage of votes by selection*

TABLE 6.6   *A 2×2 contingency table*

	Variable 2	
Variable 1	O_{11}	O_{12}
	O_{21}	O_{22}

Plotting frequencies or relative frequencies can assist interpretation. However, we should not disregard the utility of the tabular presentation of these data. Tables such as Table 6.4 are like correlation tables. As with correlation, we can ask whether the two variables in the table are independent or associated in some way. Such tables are referred to as *two-way tables* or *contingency tables*.

An important measure or statistic based on a contingency table is the *chi-square statistic* or symbolically, χ^2. The simplest form of a contingency table, given in Table 6.6, consists of four cells based on two variables, each with two categories, a 2 × 2 table.

Each cell represents the *observed cell frequency* corresponding to the *i*th row of Variable 1 and the *j*th column of Variable 2. Symbolically, we can represent the observed cell frequency as O_{ij}. The row and column totals are called *marginals*. There are situations in which we would like to compare observed frequencies with *theoretical or expected frequencies*. For example, we can compare observed frequencies (O_{ij}) with expected frequencies (E_{ij}) based on the assumption that the two categorical variables are independent. In the case where we are assuming independence, the expected cell frequencies are given by:

$$E_{ij} = \frac{R_i C_j}{N}$$

where R_i is the row total or marginal for row i, C_j is the column total or marginal for column j, N is the total number of observations.

The chi-square statistic is used in situations where a comparison of observed and expected frequencies is appropriate. This measure is defined as:

$$\chi^2 = \sum \frac{\left(O_{ij} - E_{ij}\right)^2}{E_{ij}}$$

That is, the measure is computed by finding the difference between observed and expected frequencies for each cell, squaring these values and dividing each difference by the respective expected frequency. Finally, we sum over all possible cells.

The *contingency coefficient* is a measure of association between two categorical variables. This measure is based on the chi-square statistic:

$$C = \sqrt{\frac{\chi^2}{N + \chi^2}}$$

where N is the total number of observations. Although a useful measure, the contingency coefficient has one important limitation. The value of C is dependent on the number of categories. That is, C derived from one 2×2 table can only be compared to a C value derived from another 2×2 table; we cannot compare it to a C derived from a 3×3 table.

Example 6.3: Computing the contingency coefficient

A psychologist is interested in examining the relationship between success or failure on a job and Emotional Competency (EC). One hundred employees are given an EC test. The results are presented in Table 6.7.

TABLE 6.7 Data for job performance and EC test

	EC test		
Job performance	pass	fail	Total
success	15	35	50
failure	25	25	50
Total	40	60	100

The expected frequencies are computed using the equation

$$E_{ij} = \frac{R_i C_j}{N}$$

For example, for cell (1,1) the observed value is 15. The row total R_i for row 1 is 50. The column total C_j for column 1 is 40. Therefore $E_{11} = (50 \times 40)/100 = 20$.

The χ^2 statistic is given by:

$$\chi^2 = \sum \frac{(O_{ij} - E_{ij})^2}{E_{ij}}$$

Table 6.8 sets out the computational details.

TABLE 6.8   Computational details for Table 6.7

O	E	(O_E)	$(O - E)^2$	$(O - E)^2/E$
15	20	−5	25	1.25
35	30	5	25	0.83
25	20	5	25	1.25
25	30	−5	25	0.83
100	100	0		4.17

Therefore, $\chi^2 = 4.17$.

The contingency coefficient is given by

$$C = \sqrt{\frac{\chi^2}{N + \chi^2}}$$

$$C = \sqrt{\frac{4.17}{4.17 + 100}}$$

$$C = \sqrt{0.04}$$

$$C = 0.20$$

This results in a weak relationship between successful job performance and performance on an EC test.

The chi-square statistic is one of the most important measures in statistical theory. We will return to this measure and to contingency tables.

INFERENCE: FROM SAMPLES TO POPULATIONS

In Chapter 5 we described a set of descriptive summary measures for a set of data. Those summary measures would be correct for those data, provided that they were accurate. But our interpretation of the data would be limited to that set of values. The statistical sleuth, indeed any researcher, may want to make more general statements about the variable(s) of interest that go beyond a limited set of values. A clinical psychologist may be interested in the relationship between risk-taking behaviour and parental bonding in 100 adolescents in Wollongong, Australia, and describe the 100 adolescents. But clearly, the psychologist might also like to make *general* conclusions about this relationship and whether or not it holds among *all* Australian adolescents.

Statistical inference is that part of statistics that addresses the problem of generalizing from results based on a *particular* small collection of values to *all possible observations* that may be made about a variable or variables. In Chapter 4, we used the term *population* to refer to the potential set of values for an entity of interest. This set of values can be large but finite, or it can be infinitely large. In many cases it would be impractical, indeed impossible to observe all instances of the population variable, and therefore, quite difficult to produce population summary measures. The alternative strategy is to observe only a limited set of values drawn from the population using an appropriate selection method. We refer to this subset or subgroup of values as a *sample*.

Values in a sample are only a selection from the population. It follows that summary measures such as mean and variance of a sample of values may be different from the summary measures based on population data. It is also possible that summary statistics may vary for each sample drawn from the population. None the less, each sample can be compared to the population and so can be used to draw inferences about the population. This is an important idea underlying statistical inference.

Parameters, Estimates and Statistics

Summary measures such as the mean and variance can be obtained for both populations and samples. However, a distinction needs to be made between the properties of populations and the properties of samples. We use the term *parameter* to refer to properties of populations. The mean and variance of a population are referred to as *population parameters*.

Samples are drawn from populations. Often we do not know the values of population parameters. We can obtain summary measures for a sample to say something about the population parameters. The sample measures, however, are *estimates* of the corresponding population characteristics or properties. Suppose, for example, that we sample 500 Australian males, aged between 18 and 25 years, and ask them about their weekly consumption of chocolate biscuits. Our findings yield that, on average, young males consume 15.5 chocolate biscuits per week. This mean value is an estimate of the population parameter. It is an estimate of the mean weekly consumption of chocolate biscuits we would have obtained had we been able to survey all Australian males aged between 18 and 25 years. Measures based on or derived from sample information are referred to as sample statistics.

A widely used convention is to use Greek letters to represent population parameters and Roman letters to represent sample statistics. Thus we use the Greek letter μ (pronounced mu) to represent the population mean. So far we have used the letter M, or the symbol $\bar{X}$, to represent the sample mean. Likewise, we have used the letter s to represent the sample standard deviation. We use the Greek letter σ (pronounced sigma) to represent the population standard deviation. We use the Greek letter ρ (pronounced rho) to refer to the population correlation, while the letter r symbolizes the sample correlation.

Sampling Distributions

Sample statistics are estimates of population parameters. Each sample estimate will vary from the population parameter. In other words, there is an error in estimation associated with taking any sample. This error is referred to as the *sampling error*. Sampling error will occur even with random sampling.

When we talk about sampling error we also need to talk about *sampling distributions*. For example, we could, theoretically, take all possible random samples from the population of Australian men. Each sample would then consist of N men. It is possible that we may actually have an infinite number of samples of size N.

We now compute the mean height, M, for each sample.

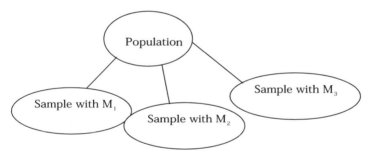

We can expect the mean of each sample to be different from each other as well as different from the population mean. Some sample means will be very different from the population mean and others will be very close to the population mean. In short, we have a range of values of M: we will have a *distribution* of sample means. We would then discover that a small number of the sample means are very different from the population. Most samples, though, will be close to the population mean. In other words, what we would have arrived at is a frequency distribution of sample means.

We might have drawn 193 samples with 20 men in each sample. We calculate the mean height for each sample. Let's look at a hypothetical frequency distribution of sample means.

Height (in cm)	Frequency
155–159	5.00
160–164	6.00
165–169	9.00
170–174	10.00
175–179	15.00
180–184	30.00
185–189	45.00
190–194	35.00
195–199	20.00
200–204	10.00
205–209	5.00
210–215	3.00

The histogram for this distribution is presented below

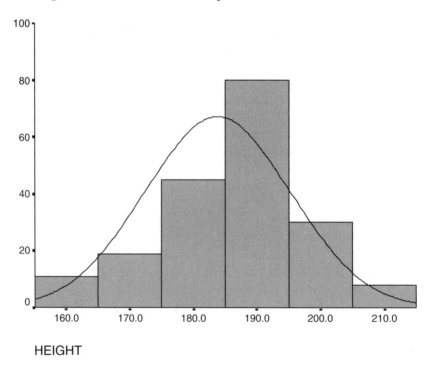

HEIGHT

An important feature of this distribution is that it appears *normally distributed*, a phrase used by statisticians to describe a curve which is symmetrical and unimodal. Heights of people, for example, tend to be normally distributed. Furthermore, we can consider the likelihood or probability of each mean value occurring. The probability that the man who is 210 cm is close to the mean of the distribution is very low. This distribution of sample means and their respective probabilities is called the *sampling distribution of the mean*. It is important to keep in mind that this is a distribution of values and therefore it is possible to find the mean and variance of this distribution.

Sampling distributions can be applied to other statistics, not just the sample mean. For example, we can consider a sampling distribution for the median. Provided that it is possible to obtain a sample statistic, then a sampling distribution for that statistic is possible.

There are three very important properties associated with the sampling distribution of the mean.

1 If we have a population with mean μ and we take random samples of size N, then the mean of the sampling distribution of sample means is equal to the population mean μ.
2 The variance of the sampling distribution of sample means will be equal to σ^2/N. That is, the variance of the sampling distribution will be equal to the population variance σ^2 divided by N, the number of observations in each sample.
3 Irrespective of the form of the population distribution, the sampling distribution of the mean will approach the normal distribution, provided that the sample size N is sufficiently large. The closer the original distribution is to the form or shape of the normal distribution, the less the requirement that N be large.

The *normal distribution* is a very important mathematical distribution in statistical theory. It is also referred to as the *normal curve*. The normal curve, as mentioned, is unimodal (has just one mode) and is symmetrical, as illustrated in Figure 6.10.

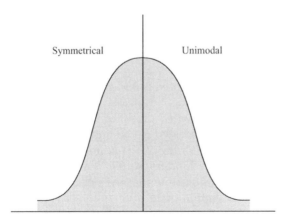

FIGURE 6.10 *The normal distribution of a normal curve*

Hypothesis Testing – Don't just show me the evidence, convince me that it is so!

We can test whether a sample comes from a population. This is hypothesis testing. To do this you will need a set of data, usually drawn from a random sample. It is also important to know something about the underlying process that generates the data – a probability model for the data. You will need to make some assertions about the population, particularly a population parameter, like the mean. These assertions or statements are referred to as *hypotheses*. There are usually two contradictory hypotheses, the *null hypothesis* (H_0) and the alternative hypothesis (H_A). The null hypothesis is tested using the data. If we did not have any data on which to base our test, then the assertion in the null hypothesis would be true.

The next step in the hypothesis-testing process involves computing one or more statistics associated with the null hypothesis. On the basis of the sample information we examine whether there is evidence supporting H_0 or refuting H_0 and supporting H_A. We retain H_0 unless there is substantial evidence to the contrary. We accept H_A if the sample data challenges the validity of H_0.

What do we mean by substantial evidence? The traditional approach is to assess the evidence against the null hypothesis using probability. How likely are we to obtain an outcome based on the sample data that is different from what we would expect if the null hypothesis were true? This probability is called the *p-value* of the test. Small p-values are evidence against the null hypothesis (Hayes, 1988).

Hypothesis testing is used to test whether the data are consistent with a *single* value of the population parameter. We might not be interested in testing just a single value but rather identifying a range of parameter values that are consistent with the data. In this case we should use an approach known as *confidence intervals*. As the name suggests, a confidence interval defines a range of values based on the sample data and the probability value α that the parameter of interest will fall within this interval. Before returning to confidence intervals, let's look at some tests for samples.

One-Sample Tests

Let's start with statistical procedures used to make inferences about populations where we have information from one sample. Imagine an anthropologist who is studying an isolated group of villagers on a remote island. As part of this study she is interested in the literacy of the young adults on the island. She measures the literacy of 100 young adults and finds that the mean literacy for the young islanders is 105. Does this sample differ from the general population? Let's assume that the population mean for literacy is 100 with a standard deviation of 15.

How do we go about answering this question? The first step is to make use of sampling distributions, in particular the sampling distribution of the mean. We know that the sample mean has a distribution approximating the normal distribution with mean μ and variance σ^2/N.

We can translate the research question set by our anthropologist into a set of hypotheses as follows:

$$H_0 : \mu = 100$$

$$H_A : \mu \neq 100$$

That is, if the null hypothesis is true then the population mean is 100.

To test the null hypothesis we use the Z-test. This test computes a Z statistic given by:

$$Z = \frac{\bar{X} - \mu_{\bar{X}}}{\sigma_{\bar{X}}}$$

where $\bar{X}$ is the sample mean, $\mu_{\bar{X}}$ is the mean of the sampling distribution of the mean and $\sigma_{\bar{X}}$ is the standard deviation of the sampling distribution of the mean. The statistic Z is distributed as a normal distribution with mean 0 and standard deviation 1. Once we have calculated Z we can look up a set of normal tables or use a computer to obtain the probability of finding a standard norm value equal to or as low as the calculated Z.

For our example we have:

$$Z = \frac{\bar{X} - \mu_{\bar{X}}}{\sigma_{\bar{X}}}$$

where $\sigma_{\bar{X}} = \sigma/\sqrt{N}$ and N is the sample size.

$$Z = \frac{105 - 100}{15/\sqrt{100}}$$

$$Z = \frac{5}{1.5}$$

$$Z = 3.33$$

The p-value associated with this Z is 0.0004. This result provides support for the alternative hypothesis rather than the null hypothesis. Our anthropologist can conclude that, in terms of literacy, her sample is different from the standard population.

If our anthropologist wishes to construct a confidence interval for the population mean, she can use the following formula:

$$\bar{X} \pm z \frac{\sigma}{\sqrt{N}}$$

TABLE 6.9 *Some commonly used values from a set of normal tables*

Confidence level	z
95%	1.96
99%	2.58

where z is the upper $(1 - \alpha)/2$ critical value for a standard normal distribution. We find these values from a set of tables. We provide some commonly used values in Table 6.9

For our data the confidence level is given by $105 - (1.96)1.5$ or between 102.06 and 107.94. That is, we can say with 95 per cent confidence that the population mean lies in the interval 102.06 and 107.94.

Often we do not have complete information on the population parameters. What are the implications for using the Z-test when the population standard deviation is unknown? It's time now to turn to history and examine the work of William Gosset.

'It's not the drink I tell you!!' 'These beer samples are not normally distributed.'

William Gosset is credited with discovering the t-distribution. The t-distribution is a very special distribution used in statistical testing. A brewery employed Gosset in Dublin as a statistician. Why employ a statistician? Gosset was required to examine the variability of beer. From a quality control point of view his task was to identify ways of maintaining variability within acceptable limits. He was hampered by two very important limits, small samples and not knowing the variability of the population parameter. So if I take the Z statistic, what happens when I replace the population parameter with an estimate of that parameter? Answer, the resulting statistic is distributed slightly differently from the normal distribution – the t-distribution in Figure 6.11. However, what is interesting about Figure 6.11 is that if the degrees of freedom increased, then the t-distribution would start to resemble the normal curve. You start to get less and less extreme scores in the tail as the sample gets bigger.

Let's consider again our anthropologist and assume that the population is unknown. In this case we cannot use the Z-test. We use a one-sample t-test. The form of the t-test is very similar to the Z-test. The only differences are that we estimate the population using the sample standard deviation and that the t-statistic is distributed as a t-distribution. The t-distribution shares many features of the normal distribution. It is unimodal and symmetrical but it is also leptokurtic, that is, it is more peaked than the normal distribution. There is also a different t-distribution for each number of degrees of freedom. *Degrees of freedom* refers to the number of values that are free to

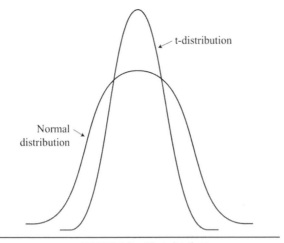

FIGURE 6.11   *The t-distribution*

vary given certain restrictions imposed on the data. For the one-sample test, the t-distribution has $N - 1$ degrees of freedom.

The t-test is given by:

$$t = \frac{\bar{X} - \mu_{\bar{X}}}{s_{\bar{X}}}$$

where $s_{\bar{X}}$ is the estimate of the standard deviation of the sampling distribution defined as $s_{\bar{X}} = s/\sqrt{N}$ where s is the standard deviation of the sample. In order to calculate $s_{\bar{X}}$ our anthropologist would need to compute the sample standard deviation and divide this value by the square root of the sample size. Once we have computed t, we can find the p-value associated with this value by consulting t-distribution tables.

The logic underlying the construction of a confidence interval for the population mean when σ is unknown is similar to that when the parameter is known. In this case, the confidence is given by

$$\bar{X} \pm ts_{\bar{X}}$$

The value of t defining either 95 or 99 per cent confidence intervals varies as the degrees of freedom vary. Consider a hypothetical example where $\bar{X} = 25.5$, $s = 7$ and $N = 16$. The degrees of freedom in this example are $N - 1 = 16 - 1$ or 15. Assume we wish to construct a 95 per cent confidence interval, then the t value with 15 degrees of freedom is 2.13. $s_{\bar{X}} = s/\sqrt{N} = 7/\sqrt{16} = 1.75$. Thus the limits of the confidence interval are $25.5 - 2.13(1.75)$ and $25.5 + 2.13(1.75)$ or 21.77 and 29.23.

One-Sample Test for Categorical Data

In 1866 the botanist and monk Gregor Mendel reported the findings of his experiments on hybridization of peas. In one experiment he observed the shape and colour of peas from a sample of plants. The hybrid plants were crossed with each other and yielded 556 seeds, of which 315 were round and yellow, 101 wrinkled and yellow, 108 round and green, and 32 wrinkled and green. His genetic theory hypothesized that the expected frequency should be in the ratio 9:3:3:1. Was he right?

Mendel's data are categorical. There are four categories of shape and colour of peas, round and yellow, wrinkled and yellow, round and green, and wrinkled and green. The null hypothesis is that the actual frequencies will equal the expected frequencies across the genotypic categories. How do we test this hypothesis? We test the null hypothesis by using the chi-square statistic discussed earlier.

Like all the statistics we have discussed so far, the chi-square has a theoretical sampling distribution that is well known. The distribution is a function of degrees of freedom. There is a different sampling distribution for each value of degrees of freedom. Furthermore, we can find a p-value for any value of chi-square. The hypothesis-testing procedure is much the same as that used with the normal and t-distributions.

Recall that the chi-square statistic is:

$$\chi^2 = \sum \frac{(O_i - E_i)^2}{E_i}$$

where O_i and E_i are the observed and expected frequencies respectively in the ith category. The expected frequencies for each cell is given by Np_i where p_i is the probability of being in the ith cell and N is the total number of observations or frequencies. The chi-square statistic has chi-square distribution with $C - 1$ degrees of freedom where C is the number of categories.

The frequencies and computations are presented in Table 6.10.

The obtained chi-square value is 0.470. The p-value associated with this value lies between 0.90 and 0.95. It follows that we have grounds for retaining the null hypothesis. In other words, the sample data support Mendel's theory.

TABLE 6.10 Frequencies in colour and shape of peas

	O_i	E_i	$(O_i - E_i)^2/E_i$
Round yellow	315	312.75	0.016
Round green	108	104.25	0.135
Wrinkled yellow	101	104.25	0.101
Wrinkled green	32	34.75	0.218
Total			0.470

Source: Ferguson, 1959: 161

Two-Sample Tests

Test of Equality of Means for Independent Samples

Social scientists like to compare groups. Do men and women differ in their attitudes to capital punishment? Do men and women differ in their voting patterns? Do students who receive one-to-one tuition perform better at statistics than students who do not? The main feature of all these questions is that they involve the comparison of two groups. In this section we describe a number of statistical tests that can be used to compare two independent groups or samples.

A sports psychologist, Dr Sam Dunk, is interested in the effectiveness of imagery as a preparation strategy on the accuracy of basketball free throws. Ten players of equal ability are randomly assigned to two conditions (five players in each condition). Players in the first condition receive no special training while the players in condition 2 are trained in mental imagery. After training each player is required to make 10 free throws; the score is the number of successful attempts. The scores are in Table 6.11.

Does imagery training affect accuracy of free throwing?

We can attempt to answer this question by examining the mean free throw score for each group. We can strengthen our argument by using the t-test for independent samples. The basic idea underlying this test is a comparison of means. If the training strategy is effective then the mean of Group 2 should be significantly different from that of Group 1. If the strategy is ineffective then the means will be similar. What we are actually doing in this case is comparing two population means, by testing the null hypothesis that the two population means are equal, $H_0 : \mu_1 = \mu_2$.

We can estimate the difference between the population means $\mu_1 - \mu_2$ using the difference between the sample means, $\bar{X}_1 - \bar{X}_2$. In order to use this statistic inferentially we need to know its sampling distribution. From this distribution we will be able to determine the probability of obtaining a difference in drawing random samples of any size. The mean of the sampling distribution of differences is equal to the difference of the population means, $\mu_1 - \mu_2$. The variance of the sampling distribution of differences, represented symbolically as $\sigma^2_{\bar{x}_1 - \bar{x}_2}$, is:

$$\sigma^2_{\bar{x}_1 - \bar{x}_2} = \frac{\sigma^2_1}{n_1} + \frac{\sigma^2_2}{n_2}$$

TABLE 6.11   *Hypothetical data for number of successful free throws in two conditions*

No training	Imagery training
6	6
4	8
5	9
5	7
5	8

where σ_1^2 and σ_2^2 are the variances of the populations. This sampling distribution will be normal. If the population variances are unknown, then we can use the sample variances to estimate the population parameters. This estimate is

$$s_{\bar{x}_1 - \bar{x}_2}^2 = \frac{s_1^2}{n_1} + \frac{s_2^2}{n_2}$$

The square root of this estimate (that is, the estimate of the standard deviation of the sampling distribution) is the *standard error* of the difference of the means. The ratio of the difference between the sample means and the estimate of the standard error is the t statistic.

$$t = \frac{\bar{X}_1 - \bar{X}_2}{s_{\bar{x}_1 - \bar{x}_2}^2}$$

In most texts this ratio is said to have a t-distribution with degrees of freedom $n_1 + n_2 - 2$. However, Moore and McCabe (1993) note that this statistic does not have a t-distribution, but rather only approximates the t-distribution. The t statistic will have a t-distribution with degrees of freedom $n_1 + n_2 - 2$ when the two population distributions have the same standard deviations. In other words, both sample variances approximate the population variance. In this case, the estimate of the standard deviation can be expressed as a weighted average of the sample variances.

$$s_p = \sqrt{\frac{(n_1 - 1)s_1^2 + (n_2 - 1)s_2^2}{n_1 + n_2 - 2}}$$

The pooled estimate assumes that the population variances are equal. This assumption is known as the *homogeneity of variance assumption*, an important assumption of the t-test for independent samples. The t statistic, when we assume that the populations have the same variances, is:

$$t = \frac{\bar{X}_1 - \bar{X}_2}{s_p \sqrt{\dfrac{1}{n_1} + \dfrac{1}{n_2}}}$$

Example 6.4: t-test for independent samples

A not so well–known Sherlock Holmes case is that of whether environmental temperature affects performance on a mental ability test. Two groups of people are randomly assigned to two conditions — a hot condition and a condition in which it is cold. Scores on the ability test are collected (high scores out of 20 indicate better performance) and the summary statistics are reported in Table 6.12. Holmes decides that a t-test for independent samples is needed!

TABLE 6.12   *Descriptive statistics*

Condition	Mean	Standard deviation	Sample size
Hot	15.5	3.25	10
Cold	12.0	2.95	10

Holmes hypothesizes that:

$$H_0 : \mu_1 - \mu_2 = 0$$

$$H_A : \mu_1 - \mu_2 \neq 0$$

Holmes should first compute s_p.

$$s_p = \sqrt{\frac{(n_1 - 1)s_1^2 + (n_2 - 1)s_2^2}{n_1 + n_2 - 2}}$$

$$s_p = \sqrt{\frac{(10 - 1)(3.25)^2 + (10 - 1)(2.95)^2}{10 + 10 - 2}}$$

$$s_p = \sqrt{\frac{173.385}{18}}$$

$$s_p = \sqrt{9.6325} = 3.1036$$

Now Holmes can compute t.

$$t = \frac{\bar{X}_1 - \bar{X}_2}{s_p\sqrt{\frac{1}{n_1} + \frac{1}{n_2}}}$$

$$t = \frac{15.5 - 12.0}{3.1036\left(\sqrt{\frac{1}{10} + \frac{1}{10}}\right)}$$

$$t = \frac{3.5}{1.388}$$

$$t = 2.52$$

Holmes notes that there are 18 degrees of freedom. The p-value for $t = 2.52$ lies between 0.05 and 0.01. He concludes that there is sufficient evidence to reject the null hypothesis. On the basis of the sample information we can say that environment does affect performance on an ability test.

Just as we define a confidence interval for the population mean, we can also define a range of values that we say will contain the difference between two population means with 95 per cent or 99 per cent confidence. If we draw a random sample of size n_1 from a population with unknown mean μ_1 and we also draw a second sample of size n_2 from a population with unknown mean μ_2, and we assume that the populations have the same variance, then we can define a 95 per cent or 99 per cent confidence interval for $\mu_1 - \mu_2$ as

$$(\bar{X}_1 - \bar{X}_2) \pm t \times s_p \sqrt{\frac{1}{n_1} + \frac{1}{n_2}}$$

The value of t comes from a t-distribution with $(n_1 + n_2 - 2)$ degrees of freedom.

From the example above, Sherlock Holmes could just as well have constructed a confidence interval for the difference of the population means. The computations are presented below:

$$(\bar{X}_1 - \bar{X}_2) \pm t \times s_p \sqrt{\frac{1}{n_1} + \frac{1}{n_2}}$$

$$= 3.5 \pm 2.10(1.388)$$

$$= 0.59 - 6.41$$

Therefore the difference between the population means will lie between 0.58 and 6.41 with 95 per cent confidence. The t-value with 18 degrees of freedom is 2.10. Recall that our null hypothesis is $H_0 : \mu_1 - \mu_2 = 0$. The value 0 (the value of the difference between the means when the null hypothesis is true) is *not* contained in this interval. Therefore we have supporting evidence to reject the null hypothesis.

If we assume that the population variances are unequal, then the confidence interval is

$$(\bar{X}_1 - \bar{X}_2) \pm t \sqrt{\frac{s_1^2}{n_1} + \frac{s_2^2}{n_2}}$$

The degrees of freedom is this case are the smaller of $n_1 - 1$ and $n_2 - 1$.

The following table presents some values of t for constructing a 95 per cent confidence interval.

df	t	df	t	df	t
1	12.71	11	2.20	25	2.06
2	4.30	12	2.18	30	2.04
3	3.18	13	2.16	40	2.02
4	2.78	14	2.15	50	2.00
5	2.58	15	2.13	60	2.00
6	2.45	16	2.12	80	1.99
7	2.37	17	2.11	100	1.98
8	2.31	18	2.10	1000	2.813
9	2.26	19	2.09		
10	2.23	20	2.09		

Based on Griffiths, Stirling, Weldon (1998)

Rank Test for Independent Samples

The statistical tests we have considered so far involve assumptions about the distributions of variables from populations. The Z and t-tests, for example, assume that the populations from which the samples are drawn are normally distributed. The statistical sleuth may on some occasions encounter situations where little is known about the population from which the sample is drawn, or where there is evidence suggesting that the population distribution is not normal. There is a family of tests that do not make assumptions about the population distribution. These tests are referred to as *distribution free* or *non-parametric*. We will now consider a test for two independent samples. This test uses the ranks of values rather than the actual scores. Therefore, it is usually referred to as a rank test.

In the rank test we would assume that a person has been randomly assigned to a particular group. Assume for the moment that people are not assigned to groups and we assume a rank, r_i, to each of the scores, x_{ij}. Next we return the scores to their original group. If the groups are different, then the sum of the ranks or the average ranks for each group will be different for each group. If the groups have similar scores then the average ranks or sum of the ranks will be similar. Denote the sum of the ranks as R_1 and R_2 respectively. We can test whether the groups are different by applying the Mann-Whitney U test. We compute two values U_1 and U_2:

$$U_1 = n_1 n_2 + \frac{n_1(n_1 + 1)}{2} - R_1$$

$$U_2 = n_1 n_2 + \frac{n_2(n_2 + 1)}{2} - R_2$$

where n_1 and n_2 refer to the number of observations in groups 1 and 2 respectively. We calculate a statistic U to be the smaller of U_1 and U_2.

The Mann-Whitney U test is used with small samples. For large samples we can compute a z statistic defined as follows:

$$z = \frac{U - n_1 n_2/2}{\sqrt{\dfrac{n_1 n_2 (n+1)}{12}}}$$

where n is the total number of observations. Once we have calculated this value we can find the p-value associated with it. In the case of tied ranks the formula for z is slightly different.

$$z = \frac{U - (n_1 n_2/2)}{\sqrt{\left(\dfrac{n_1 n_2}{n^2 - n}\right)\left(\dfrac{n^3 - n}{12}\right) - \sum T}}$$

where $T = (t^3 - t)/12$, and t is the number of tied values.

Example 6.5: Rank test for two independent groups

Consider the following observations for two samples.

Sample 1: 44 32 38 51 54 56 67 69 62 73

Sample 2: 6 10 13 14 29 42 26 46 50 55 70 77

We wish to test the hypothesis that the samples come from different populations. We can use the test

$$z = \frac{U - n_1 n_2/2}{\sqrt{\dfrac{n_1 n_2 (n+1)}{12}}}$$

to test this hypothesis. The first step is to rank-order the values and obtain the following ranks.

Sample 1: 10 7 8 13 14 16 18 19 17 21

Sample 2: 1 2 3 4 6 9 5 11 12 15 20 22

In order to compute U we need to compute U_1 and U_2.

$$U_1 = n_1 n_2 + \frac{n_1 (n_1 + 1)}{2} - R_1$$

$$U_2 = n_1 n_2 + \frac{n_2(n_2 + 1)}{2} - R_2$$

The sum of the ranks for sample 1 R_1 is 143, while the sum of ranks for sample 2 R_2 is 110. n_1 and n_2 are 10 and 12 respectively.

$$U_1 = n_1 n_2 + \frac{n_1(n_1 + 1)}{2} - R_1$$

$$U_2 = n_1 n_2 + \frac{n_2(n_2 + 1)}{2} - R_2$$

$$U_1 = 10(12) + 10(11)/2 - 143$$

$$U_1 = 32$$

$$U_2 = 10(12) + 12(13)/2 - 110$$

$$U_2 = 88$$

U is defined as the smaller of U_1 and U_2. So $U = 32$. We now need to find z.

$$z = \frac{U - nn_2/2}{\sqrt{\frac{n_1 n_2(n + 1)}{12}}}$$

$$z = \frac{32 - 10(12)/2}{\sqrt{\frac{10(12)(22 + 1)}{12}}}$$

$$z = \frac{-28}{\sqrt{230}}$$

$$z = -1.85$$

The p-value associated with z is 0.0322. On the basis of this evidence we can retain the alternative hypothesis. There is evidence that the samples come from different populations.

Tests for Categorical Data

Guilford (1965: 234) cited the work of Baller (1936) who reported a study that examined whether intelligence level was contingent on marital status. The study reports two samples of 206 young American males. The men in the first sample were regarded as feeble-minded in terms of IQ when they were in school. The second group of men of similar age had IQ levels in the normal range. The cross-tabulation of marital status and intelligence is presented in Table 6.13.

TABLE 6.13   Frequencies relating to marital status and IQ

	Feeble-minded	Normal	Total
Married	84	111	195
Unmarried	122	95	217
Total	206	206	412

You will recall that this is a two-way table or a contingency table. These tables are useful for displaying the cell frequencies for two categorical variables. We can examine the cell frequencies and surmise whether one variable is related to or independent of the second. Baller noted that the proportions of married men were 0.408 and 0.539 for 'feeble minded' and normal categories respectively. Is this difference in proportions in marital status statistically significant? To examine these questions we use the chi-square statistic we introduced earlier in this chapter. The statistic is

$$\chi^2 = \sum \frac{\left(O_{ij} - E_{ij}\right)^2}{E_{ij}}$$

Under the null hypothesis of independence the expected cell frequencies are equal to:

$$E_{ij} = \frac{R_i C_j}{N}$$

where R_i is the row total or marginal for row i, C_j is the column total or marginal for column j, N is the total number of observations. The chi-square statistic has a chi-square distribution with $(r-1)(c-1)$ degrees of freedom where r is the number of rows and c is the number of columns. In the case of Baller's data the degrees of freedom are $(2-1)(2-1) = 1$. Once we have calculated the statistic we can find its corresponding p-value.

For Baller's data we have in Table 6.14 a comparison of observed and expected frequencies.

You can see from this table that, for each cell, we compute the value $(O-E)^2/E$ and then sum these values across the cells. The obtained chi-square statistic is 7.10 in this case. The p-value associated with this

TABLE 6.14   Comparison of observed and expected frequencies for Baller's data

Cell	O	E	$(O-E)$	$(O-E)^2$	$(O-E)^2/E$
Married, feeble-minded	84	97.5	13.5	182.25	1.87
Married, normal	111	97.5	−13.5	182.25	1.87
Unmarried, feeble-minded	122	108.5	−13.5	182.25	1.68
Unmarried, normal	95	108.5	13.5	182.25	1.68
					7.10

statistic lies between 0.01 and 0.001. This result then supports the hypothesis that married and unmarried differ significantly with respect to IQ!! Of course, the statistical sleuth would ask if there is another explanation for this result. Is there another variable that may be influencing the frequencies? It is possible to examine the relationship among three or more categorical variables simultaneously. The chi-square test for independence cannot be used to examine more than two variables. If the researcher wished to look at the interaction of three or more categorical variables then he or she would need to refer to what are called log-linear models. Howell (1992) and Agresti (1990) give excellent introductory accounts of these techniques.

Tests for Related Samples

We have discussed methods of comparing samples that are independent of each other. Although the research design that generates these data is common in the social sciences, we may also wish to use research designs which generate data about the sample over time. For example, a statistics lecturer may be interested in comparing performance on statistical problems at different times of the day. He chooses two problems of equal difficulty. One problem is given to students in the morning, the other problem is given in the afternoon. That is, the same student completes each problem. This is an example of a *within-subjects design*.

Consider a psychologist who is interested in the effectiveness of a treatment for speech anxiety. Twenty volunteers agree to participate in the study. All participants are initially tested for level of speech anxiety. On the basis of this test 10 pairs of participants are identified where each member of the pair has the same level of speech anxiety. One member of the pair is assigned to a treatment condition and the other member of the pair to a placebo condition. Each participant is then tested again on a speech anxiety measure. Although the participants are assigned to different conditions, they are still correlated or *matched* on initial level of anxiety. How does our researcher test for group differences?

The data obtained from the designs can be analysed using a technique called a related samples t-test. Consider N pairs of observations (X_i, X_j). They might be two people paired or matched in terms of anxiety scores or the observations may be paired because one observation has been taken in the morning, the other in the afternoon. We can find the difference between any pair of observations (X_i, X_j), and we will denote this difference as $D = X_i - X_j$. Furthermore, we can find the mean, $\bar{D}$, of these differences. As with other tests of significance we have discussed in this chapter, the statistic $\bar{D}$ has a sampling distribution. The estimate of the variance of the sampling distribution of $\bar{D}$ is

$$s_{\bar{D}}^2 = \frac{s_D^2}{N}$$

where s_D^2 is the variance of the Ds:

TABLE 6.15   *Hypothetical data for speech anxiety scores in two conditions*

Treatment condition	Placebo
23	24
20	26
24	27
26	22
18	20
19	19
17	20
15	25
25	21
21	27

$$s_D^2 = \frac{\sum D^2 - \left(\sum D\right)^2 / N}{N - 1}$$

We can define the t statistic:

$$t = \frac{\bar{D}}{s_D}$$

$$t = \frac{\bar{D}}{\sqrt{s_D^2 / N - 1}}$$

This statistic is distributed as a t-distribution with $N - 1$ degrees of freedom. We should remember that the numerator of the t statistic is in fact $\bar{D} - 0$. Let's return to one of our examples to see how this test is applied.

Consider again the psychologist who is interested in speech anxiety. The scores on the anxiety test are in Table 6.15.

Our researcher hypothesizes that the two groups will differ in level of anxiety. The null hypothesis then is $H_0 : \mu_1 - \mu_2 = 0$. That is, the difference in the population means is zero.

In order to apply the t-test we need to compute D.

Treatment condition	Placebo	D	D²
23	24	−1	1
20	26	−6	36
24	27	−3	9
26	22	4	16
18	20	−2	4
19	19	0	0
17	20	−3	9
15	25	−10	100
25	21	4	16
21	27	−6	36

We find the $\bar{D} = -23/10 = -2.3$. The variance of D is

$$s_D^2 = \frac{\sum D^2 - \left(\sum D\right)^2 / N}{N - 1}$$

$$s_D^2 = \frac{227 - (-23)^2 / 10}{10 - 1}$$

$$s_D^2 = 19.344$$

We now compute t:

$$t = \frac{\bar{D}}{\sqrt{S_D^2 / N}}$$

$$t = \frac{-2.3}{\sqrt{19.344 / 10}}$$

$$t = -1.654$$

This t statistic is distributed as a t-distribution with $N - 1 = 9$ degrees of freedom. The p-value associated with this obtained t statistic lies between 0.10 and 0.20. On this evidence we should retain the null hypothesis and conclude that the treatment has not affected speech anxiety.

Rank Test for Correlated or Related Samples
The Wilcoxon signed ranks test is a distribution-free alternative to the t-test for related samples. This test is based not on the difference between pairs of scores, but rather the ranks of the differences. Difference scores are ranked with respect to their magnitude, but not their sign (whether they are positive or negative). Once we have ranked the difference scores we re-assign the signs, and compute the sum of the positive difference scores, T_1, and the sum of the negative difference scores, T_2. We now compute a statistic T that is the smaller of T_1 and T_2. There are 2^N possible signed ranks in this example. Assuming that each pair of scores is random, then each of the 2^N sets of ranks is equally likely. Consider the case where N is 5. In this case we have 32 sets of possible ranks. The probability that T_1 is zero is $1/32$, the probability that T_1 is 1 is also $1/32$. The probability that T_1 is either 0 or 1 is $2/32$. This pattern is also the same for T_2. Furthermore, the probability that either T_1 or T_2 is 0 is $2/32$. It is therefore possible to

construct a table of probabilities for any sample size – this is the sampling distribution for T (Roscoe, 1975).

Under the null hypothesis of no difference between groups, one would anticipate that T_1 and T_2 would be the same. In this case the value of T would be maximal. However, if the groups are different, then there will be a tendency for either T_1 to be greater than T_2 or vice versa. T will tend to be smaller and equal 0 when the two samples are maximally different.

To see how the Wilcoxon signed rank test is applied let's consider the speech anxiety example discussed earlier. Recall that we are hypothesizing that the two distributions are the same under the null. A table of difference scores and their ranks is provided below.

D	Rank of D	Pos	Neg
−1	1		1
−6	7.5		7.5
−3	3.5		3.5
4	5.5	5.5	
−2	2		2
0			
−3	3.5		3.5
−10	9		9
4	5.5	5.5	
−6	7.5		7.5

T_1 is 11 and T_2 is 34. Note that on one the difference score is 0. We do not count zero differences; we also reduce N by the number of zero differences. For this example N is now 9. T is the smaller of T_1 and T_2; T is 11. For $N = 9$ the p-value is greater than 0.05. Therefore there is evidence to retain the null. The two distributions are similar. We arrive at a similar result to the related samples t-test.

USING SPSS AND EXCEL: ONE-SAMPLE TESTS

Let's see how we can use SPSS and Excel to do one-sample tests. Let's again use Patrick Rawstorne's computer anxiety data, provided in *The Statistical Inquirer*. Patrick's data in the data file were collected from 60 undergraduate students. Assume that the mean population age of undergraduate students in Australia is 24. We can test whether the sample in this data file comes from this population.

Using SPSS we select *One-Sample T-Test* from the *Compare Means* option in the *Analyze* menu.

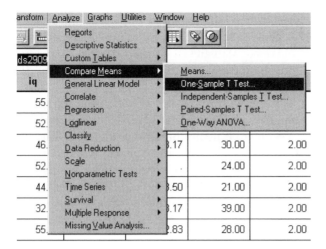

This selection will produce the One-Sample T Test dialog box.

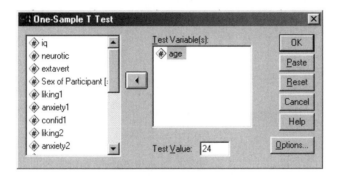

We select the variable *Age* and move it to the test variable(s) window and type the value 24 in the *Test Value* window. Click *OK* to run the procedure. Selected output from this procedure is presented below.

One-Sample Test

					95% Confidence Interval of the Difference	
	t	df	Sig. (2-tailed)	Mean Difference	Lower	Upper
AGE	1.361	59	0.179	1.6167	−0.7610	3.9943

Test Value = 24

This output gives us the t statistic, which is 1.361, and its corresponding p-value of 0.179. Convention is to reject the null hypothesis when the p-value of the obtained statistic is less than 0.05. This result provides support for the null hypothesis that the sample is from a population with mean 24.

We can conduct a one-sample z-test in Excel using the function ZTEST. Earlier in this chapter we noted that when the population variance is unknown we can estimate it using the sample variance. The resulting statistic is only distributed as a normal distribution when the sample size is large. Otherwise the new statistic is distributed as a t-distribution. SPSS does not offer a z-test for population means. The reader should note that the ZTEST function should be used with large samples when the population variance is unknown. Running the function ZTEST is quite straightforward.

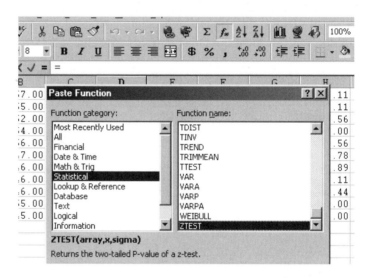

Click on the *Paste Function* button located at the top of the Excel window. Select *Statistical* from the *Function Category* window and *ZTEST* from the *Function name* window. This will produce a ZTEST dialog box.

In the *Array* window you will need to define the cell range containing the data for the variable AGE. In the X window we insert the test value (population mean) 24. The third window Sigma refers to the population standard deviation. If it is known, the user can insert the value in this window. If this window is left blank, the sample standard deviation will be used. Note that the p-value is 0.0839. On the basis of this result we retain the null hypothesis. The sample comes from a population with mean 24.

In this chapter we also discussed the chi-square test for goodness of fit – a one-sample test for categorical data. In Excel we could use the function CHITEST to conduct such a test. However, the function requires that the user provide the actual and expected cell frequencies in an Excel worksheet in order to conduct the test.

Conducting the goodness of fit chi-square test using SPSS is less complicated. One of the variables in the computer anxiety data is the average time spent on a computer. This variable is categorical, with six categories: Almost never, Less than 30 mins, from 30 mins to 60 mins, 1–2 hours, 2–3 hours, and More than 3 hours. Let's test the hypothesis that the expected frequencies will be equally distributed over the categories. To run this test in SPSS we select Chi-square from the *Nonparametric* option in the *Analyze* menu.

This will open the Chi-square test dialog box.

We select the variable of interest and move it to the *Test Variable List* window. Notice that under *Expected values* there are two radio buttons, one labelled 'All categories equal' and the other labelled 'Values'. To test our hypothesis we leave the default option 'All categories equal'. It is possible to specify the theoretical frequencies by clicking on the *Values*

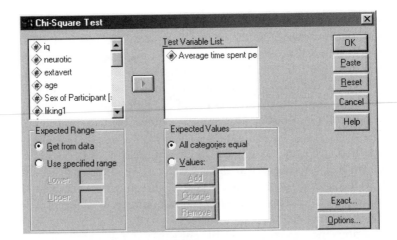

option, entering the values one at the time, and remembering to click on *Add* after each entry. To run the procedure click *OK*. The output will look as follows:

Average time spent per day

	Observed N	Expected N	Residual
Almost never	1	10.0	−9.0
Less than 30 mins.	7	10.0	−3.0
From 30 mins to 60 mins	22	10.0	12.0
1–2 hours	21	10.0	11.0
2–3 hours	4	10.0	−6.0
More than 3 hours	5	10.0	−5.0
Total	60		

Test Statistics

	Average time spent per day
Chi-Square[a]	41.600
df	5
Asymp. Sig.	0.000

[a] 0 cells (0.0%) have expected frequencies less than 5.
The minimum expected cell frequency is 10.0

The first output window gives observed and expected frequencies. The second output window gives us the obtained chi-square value (which is 41.6 in this case), the degrees of freedom and the p-value. Note that the p-value is 0.000. We have support for rejection of the null hypothesis and concluding that the responses are not equally distributed across the categories of our variable.

USING SPSS AND EXCEL: TWO-SAMPLE TESTS

We will use the *Accounting for Tastes* dataset, *tastes.sav,* in order to show how SPSS and Excel can be used for comparing two population means. We will start with a t-test for two independent samples. The hypothesis we wish to test is whether males and females differ in terms of their annual incomes. To test this hypothesis using SPSS we click on the menu *Analyze*, select *Compare means* and then choose the option *Independent Samples T Tests*.

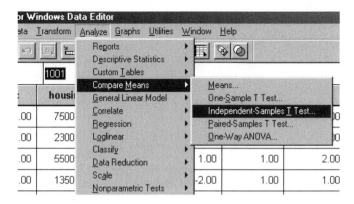

This option will open the following dialog box.

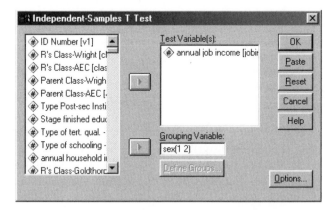

As with most procedures in SPSS we select the variable of interest, in this case 'jobinc', and move it to the *Test Variable(s)* window. Next we select the variable 'sex' and move it the *Grouping Variable* window. You need to click on the *Define Groups* button, opening the following window.

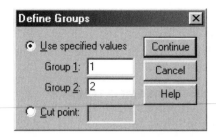

Given that Sex is coded 1 for females and 2 for males, we insert the value 1 in the *Group 1* window and 2 in the *Group 2* window. Click *Continue* followed by *OK* to run the procedure. The following output will be produced.

Group Statistics

	SEX	N	Mean	Std. Deviation	Std. Error Mean
Annual job income	1.00	1405	14052.06	15208.8114	405.7487
	2.00	1313	27427.44	22989.0154	634.4363

Independent Samples Test

		Levene's Test for Equality of Variances		t-test for Eq		
		F	Sig.	t	df	Sig. (2-tailed)
Annual job income	Equal variances assumed	131.784	0.000	−17.998	2716	0.000
	Equal variances not assumed			−17.761	2252.592	0.000

From this output we see the mean annual incomes for females (sex = 1) and males (sex = 2). In the output table titled 'Independent Samples Test', we first note that the test for homogeneity of variance (known as Levene's test) is significant. This indicates that population variances are different. The t statistic in this case is −17.761 with a p-value of 0.000. We reject the null hypothesis of equality of population means and conclude that the mean annual incomes of males and females are different. By looking at the means we see that males earn more than females.

If we assume that the data violate distributional assumptions (population distributions are not normally distributed), then we would use a non-parametric test instead of the traditional t-test to test whether the distributions for annual income differ for males and females. To conduct this test using SPSS we select *2 Independent Samples* from the *Nonparametric Tests* option in the *Analyze* menu.

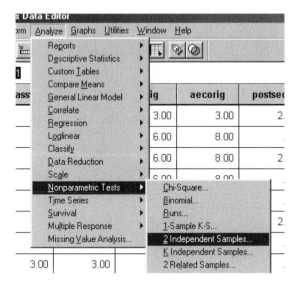

This opens a dialog box similar to that in the case of the independent samples t-test.

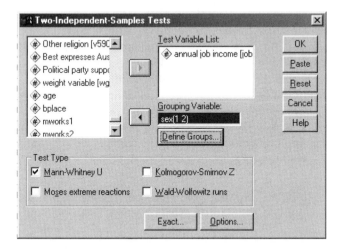

We select the dependent variable and place it in the *Test Variables* window, select the independent variable and place it in the *Grouping Variables* window and define each level of the groups as before. Note that the *Test Type* has been checked as Mann-Whitney U, which is the test we wish to conduct. Click *OK* to conduct the test. The output is shown below.

Ranks

	SEX	N	Mean Rank	Sum of Ranks
Annual job income	1.00	1405	1119.30	1572610.00
	2.00	1313	1616.54	2122511.00
	Total	2718		

Test Statistics[a]

	Annual job income
Mann-Whitney U	584895.00
Wilcoxon W	1572610.0
Z	−16.556
Asymp. Sig. (2-tailed)	0.000

[a] Grouping Variable: SEX

The first table presents the mean and sum of the ranks. In the second table we have the Mann-Whitney U statistic, the z statistic and the p-value associated with the z. The p-value is very small, providing support for rejecting the null hypothesis. Men, on average, earn more than women.

To illustrate using Excel to perform the two-sample test, we will return to the computer anxiety dataset. In this case we may be interested in investigating whether males and females differ in terms of computer anxiety. We select the *Data Analysis* option from the *Tools* menu and then select *t-test: Two-sample Assuming Equal Variances*. In the next dialog box you will need to insert the cell ranges defining the data for the males and females respectively. In this dataset we have a single variable for 'anxiety1', the computer anxiety measure, and a variable 'sex' defining the gender of each case. The data for the males is located in the first 23 rows, the data for the females in the next 37 rows. When the cell ranges have been defined, click *OK* to run the procedure.

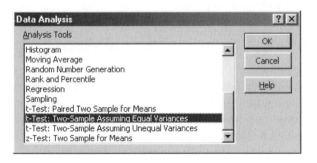

t-Test: Two-Sample Assuming Equal Variances ? X

Input
Variable 1 Range: $H$2:$H$24
Variable 2 Range: $H$25:$H$61

OK
Cancel
Help

Hypothesized Mean Difference:

☐ Labels

Alpha: 0.05

Output options
○ Output Range:
◉ New Worksheet Ply:
○ New Workbook

The output is presented below.

A	B	C
t-Test: Two-Sample Assuming Equal Variances		
	Variable 1	*Variable 2*
Mean	2.194565217	2.545945946
Variance	0.83499753	0.761996997
Observations	23	37
Pooled Variance	0.789686854	
Hypothesized Mean Difference	0	
df	58	
t Stat	-1.489154093	
P(T<=t) one-tail	0.070932306	
t Critical one-tail	1.671553491	
P(T<=t) two-tail	0.141864611	
t Critical two-tail	2.001715984	

We can see that the output contains the mean and variance for males (variable 1 in the output) and females (variable 2). The t statistic (-1.489) is also presented along with its p-value (0.071). Convention requires that the p-value be less than 0.05 in order to reject the null hypothesis. In this case, the p-value is greater than 0.05, so we retain the null.

Comparing the means of two related samples is quite simple in SPSS. Students in the computer anxiety study were tested twice on the variable 'anxiety1'. Data for time 2 computer anxiety is labelled 'anxiety2'. In other words, the scores for 'anxiety1' and 'anxiety2' are correlated because it is the same person responding twice.

In order to run a related samples t-test we select the *Paired-Samples T Test* from the *Compare Means* option in the *Analyze* menu.

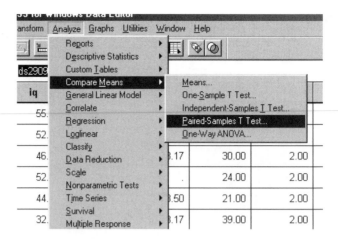

In the *Paired-Samples T-Test* dialog box we select the pair of variables we wish to analyse.

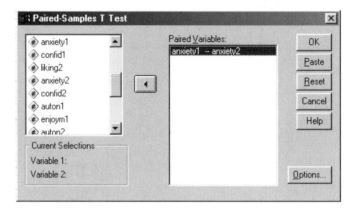

We select 'anxiety1' and 'anxiety2' and then click on the arrow button to move this pair of variables to the *Paired Variables* window. Click *OK* to run the procedure. The output generated by this procedure is presented below.

Paired Samples Test

| | | | Paired Differences | | | | |
| | | | 95% Confidence Interval of the Difference | | | | |
Mean	Std. Deviation	Std. Error Mean	Lower	Upper	t	df	Sig. (2-tailed)
060E-02	0.4332	5.689E-02	−3.33E-02	0.1945	1.417	57	0.162

As you can see, this output provides the t-value and the p-value associated with the t statistic. The p-value is large; we retain the null hypothesis and conclude that computer anxiety has not changed over time.

The Wilcoxon signed rank test is the non-parametric equivalent of the related samples t-test. To run the Wilcoxon test we select *2 Related Samples.*

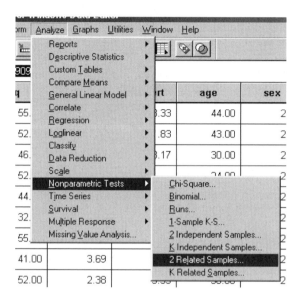

This step opens the following dialog box.

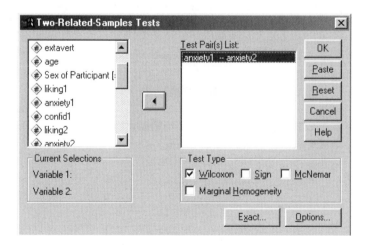

We select the pair of variables in the same way as we did with the parameter test and move them to the *Test Pair(s) List.* Click on *OK* to run the procedure. The output is presented below.

Ranks

		N	Mean Rank	Sum of Ranks
ANXIETY2 – ANXIETY1	Negative Ranks	33^a	27.73	915.00
	Positive Ranks	21^b	27.14	570.00
	Ties	4^c		
	Total	58		

[a] ANXIETY2 < ANXIETY1
[b] ANXIETY2 > ANXIETY1
[c] ANXIETY1 = ANXIETY2

Test Statistics[b]

	ANXIETY2 – ANXIETY1
Z	-1.488^a
Asymp. Sig. (2-tailed)	0.137

[a] Based on positive ranks.
[b] Wilcoxon Signed Ranks Test

The mean and sum of ranks are presented, along with the z statistic and its p-value. As we can see, the p-value is large and consequently we retain the null hypothesis – men and women do not differ in terms of computer anxiety.

We can use SPSS to test the independence of two categorical variables. With the computer anxiety data we can test whether responses on the frequency of computer use differ across males and females.

We begin by selecting cross-tabs from *Descriptive Statistics* from the *Analyze* menu.

We select the variable 'sex' and place it in the *Row(s)* window, and move the variable 'Use' (Frequency of Use) to the *Column(s)* window.

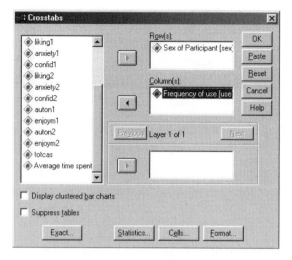

By clicking on the *Statistics* button we can choose to compute the Chi-square statistic along with a number of other measures of association for categorical data, including the contingency coefficient.

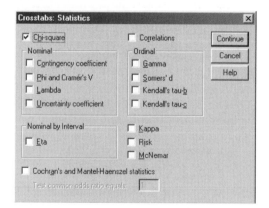

By clicking on the *Cells* button we can select an number of options, including obtaining expected and observed cell frequencies.

Click *Continue* and then *OK* to obtain the following output.

In the first table we have the observed and expected cell frequencies. In the second table we have the chi-square statistic and its associated p-value (called Pearson Chi-square in the output). This p-value is smaller than the conventional 0.05; we can conclude that the two variables are related. We also obtained row percentages and from these percentages we can see that males tend to spend more time using computers than females.

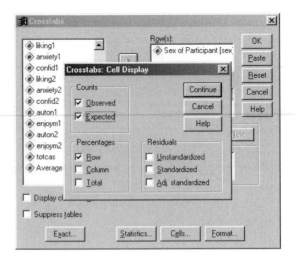

Sex of Participant * Frequency of use Crosstabulation

| | | | \multicolumn{4}{c}{Frequency of use} | | |
			A few times a month	A few times a week	About once a day	Several times a day	Total
Sex of Participant	Female	Count	2	24	7	4	37
		Expected Count	3.1	17.9	9.9	6.2	37.0
		% within Sex Participant	5.4%	64.9%	18.9%	10.8%	100.0%
	Male	Count	3	5	9	6	23
		Expected Count	1.9	11.1	6.1	3.8	23.0
		% within Sex Participant	13.0%	21.7%	39.1%	26.1%	100.0%
Total		Count	5	29	16	10	60
		Expected Count	5.0	29.0	16.0	10.0	60.0
		% within Sex Participant	8.3%	48.3%	26.7%	16.7%	100.0%

Chi-Square Tests

	Value	df	Asymp. Sig (2-sided)
Pearson Chi-Square	10.609[a]	3	0.014
Likelihood Ratio	11.098	3	0.011
Linear-by-Linear Association	3.460	1	0.063
N of Valid Cases	60		

[a] 3 cells (37.5%) have expected count less than 5. The minimum expected count is 1.92

We can use Excel to conduct a related samples t-test. Let's again use the variables 'anxiety1' and 'anxiety2'. Go to the *Tools* menu and select *Data Analysis*. We then select *t-Test: Paired Two Sample for Means*.

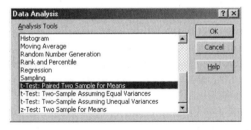

Once we have chosen the option from the Data Analysis window, it will open the next dialog box.

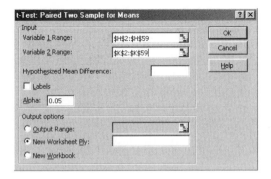

We define the cell ranges for each variable in the usual way and then click *OK*.

In our discussion on the goodness of fit chi-square statistic we mentioned we could use the CHITEST function to conduct that test. This function can also be used to test the independence of two categorical variables. We have opted not to illustrate this procedure, for the same reasons given in the one-sample case.

INTRODUCTION TO RANDOMIZATION TESTS

In recent times, there has been an increasing interest in exploring alternative approaches to computing statistical significance in cases where there is evidence that the population distributions are not normal or the random sampling assumption has been violated. The techniques underlying these approaches are not new (see Edgington, 1964, for example). The resurgence in interest is due in part to the speed with which modern desktop computers can process quite computationally intensive techniques. In particular, randomization tests have gained popularity. Randomization tests are computationally intensive, but they do not require the assumption that samples are randomly sampled.

With the tests we have considered in this chapter, we derived a p-value for a test statistic by comparing it to its sampling distribution when the null hypothesis is true. These sampling distributions are theoretical, and to use them appropriately we need to ensure that certain assumptions are met – normality assumptions, homogeneity of variance assumptions, to name but two. The idea underlying randomization tests is to construct an empirical distribution for the statistic based on permutations of the data. The number of permutations possible will in part be determined by the research design. Sometimes the number of permutations is very large and we choose a random sample of permutations to construct our permutation distribution.

Hypothesis testing with randomization tests is similar to 'traditional' testing – tests based on normal theory. The decision to retain or reject the null hypothesis is based on determining whether the obtained statistic or a value that is more extreme under the null hypothesis is uncommon.

We will use an example from May and Hunter (1993) to illustrate the logic of randomization tests. Assume we have two samples, with values 4, 5, 6 in one sample and 1, 2, 3 in the second sample. The mean of the first sample is 5.00; the mean of the second sample is 2.00. We are interested in seeing whether the means of these samples are different.

We begin by obtaining all possible permutations of the six scores 1, 2, 3, 4, 5, and 6 into two samples. We then compute the test statistic for each permutation – the mean difference. The results of these steps are presented in Table 6.16.

TABLE 6.16   All possible permutations of six scores in two conditions

Permutation	Sample 1	Sample 2	Statistic: $M_1 - M_2$
1	1,2,3	4,5,6	−3.00
2	1,2,4	3,5,6	−2.34
3	1,3,4	2,5,6	−1.66
4	1,2,5	3,4,6	−1.66
5	1,2,6	3,4,5	−1.00
6	1,3,5	2,4,6	−1.00
7	2,3,4	1,5,6	−1.00
8	1,3,6	2,4,5	−0.33
9	1,4,5	2,3,6	−0.33
10	2,3,5	1,4,6	−0.33
11	2,3,6	1,4,5	0.33
12	2,4,5	1,3,6	0.33
13	1,4,6	2,3,5	0.33
14	1,5,6	2,3,4	1.00
15	2,4,6	1,3,5	1.00
16	3,4,5	1,2,6	1.00
17	2,5,6	1,3,4	1.66
18	3,4,6	1,2,5	1.66
19	3,5,6	1,2,4	2.34
20	4,5,6	1,2,3	3.00

Source: May and Hunter, 1993

TABLE 6.17 *Permutation distribution for data in Table 6.16*

$M_1 - M_2$	f	p	Cumulative p
−3.00	1	0.05	1.00
−2.34	1	0.05	0.95
−1.66	2	0.10	0.90
−1.00	3	0.15	0.80
−0.33	3	0.15	0.65
0.33	3	0.15	0.50
1.00	3	0.15	0.35
1.66	2	0.10	0.20
2.34	1	0.05	0.10
3.00	1	0.05	0.05

Source: May and Hunter, 1993

From this table we can construct frequency and relative frequency distributions for the possible values of $M_1 - M_2$, the difference between the two sample means. The permutation distribution for these data is presented in Table 6.17.

This distribution is an 'empirically-derived' sampling distribution. We can use it to determine the 'p-value' for a value of a statistic. We can see that for a mean difference of 3 the p-value is 0.05.

For a thorough treatment of randomization tests, we refer the reader to Edgington (1995), Manly (1991) and May and Hunter (1993). There are a number of commercially available packages and freeware programs for conducting randomization tests. A brief review of these programs is presented by Hayes (1998). Hayes also presents some SPSS procedures for randomization tests.

GREAT SOCIAL BIOLOGY DETECTIVE STORIES: 'WE MUST HUNT FOR CASES'

The statistical equations that we have introduced to you are general measures, nomothetic measures, that assume that the data, the individual cases, form into patterns or distributions that are meaningful. But we have to be very careful not to impose order on data where there is none or to assume that distributions themselves create social or psychological order.

Income, for example, may form a normal distribution in a study, but it does not follow that the distribution became that way because of a normal curve. We look for patterns in the data and statistical measures assist us with interpreting those patterns.

Early work on statistics, including the use of statistics in sociology, reflected this tension between *finding order* and *imposing order*. Sociologists and psychologists, for example, have long been interested in the role of social or hereditary factors in influencing behaviour. Some of the most famous statistical measures were developed and applied in pursuit of fanciful ideas about the possibility of a 'super race', how genetics determines social order. Others, like Durkheim, were interested in statistics for the reverse reason, how social order determines behaviour.

Is There An Ideal Person?: Quetelet, Galton, Pearson

The normal distribution is attributed to Gauss and Laplace, but Adolph Quetelet carried out an early application of the normal distribution to social and biological data. Quetelet was a great promoter of the use of statistical methods in Europe. He encouraged the use of accurate statistical records for social phenomena such as births and deaths and crimes, as well as weather.

Quetelet found that the heights of French conscripts could be described using the normal curve. The normal curve suggested to Quetelet the possibility of what he called the ideal observation, the mean, and the fact that some observations deviated from this ideal. Quetelet came up with the idea of the *l'homme moyen*, the average person as nature's ideal (see Hankins, 1968).

But it is not clear that Quetelet's research on biology can simply be translated to sociology and psychology. To what extent can the normal distribution be described as a model for the variability of social and psychological phenomena? To what extent is the normal distribution a 'natural' model of social and psychological data? The idea of the normal curve has become so common in the modern research language that it is almost a given. However, even statisticians such as Karl Pearson (who reported in *Biometrika* in 1903 that cranial widths demonstrated the characteristics of a normal curve) cautioned against the universal application of the normal distribution. 'The reader may well ask ... is it not possible to find material which obeys within probable limits the normal law? I reply, yes, but *this law is not a universal law of nature. We must hunt for cases* [emphasis added]' (cited in Yule and Kendall, 1937: 186).

Let's look at some theorists who hunted for cases. Galton argued along evolutionary grounds that most human individual differences were inherited. He proposed the science of eugenics and the possibility of creating a super race through genetic manipulation. Galton set up a battery of tests. He was fanatical about counting and measuring. Some of the variables he measured in his 'anthropometric laboratory' included height, arm span, swiftness of blow and colour discrimination.

Galton had data for well over 9,000 individuals. He needed some way of summarizing these data, and in particular, summaries that would support his hereditarian hypothesis. He wanted to demonstrate the degree of similarity of measures between brothers and unrelated persons. He created scatter plots of bivariate data and identified a near straight-line relationship. Galton set the seeds for the development of the correlation coefficient and simple linear regression.

The concept of regression, or reversion, as Galton first called it, began with his work with non-human material. Galton's work started with breeding sweet peas. He started weighing thousands of pea seeds and selecting different weights. He also started measuring their diameters, which he found to be proportional to their weights. Galton sent samples of seeds varying in weights to colleagues to plant. The results of his research were reported in 1877 and suggested that the daughter seeds were not as extreme as the parent seeds. The seeds had 'reverted' to the average type of the parent seed.

Galton noted that for every unit increase in the parent seed, there was on average only a one-third increase in the unit size of the offspring seeds. This observation was the genesis of the concept known as regression towards the mean.

It was the application of this concept to human data that was of most interest to Galton. He began the human side of his investigation with the heights of parents and their children. He plotted the data, as we noted earlier in this chapter. He found that the human offspring tended to regress toward the mean, much in the same way that seed offspring did.

Galton then took the mean heights of parents and plotted this against the heights of their children. He found that he could draw a line through the scatter of points on his plot. This, of course, was the beginning of the regression line. Galton found that children of taller parents were not as tall on average as their parents, and children of shorter parents were not as short. But this finding was somewhat paradoxical. It appeared not to support the idea of full hereditary transmission of human characteristics and qualities.

Does a General Intelligence Factor Exist?: Spearman and the introduction of correlation

Charles Spearman made use of the correlation coefficient to propose a two-factor theory of intelligence. Guilford (1954: 472) stated that 'No single event in the history of mental testing has proved to be of such momentous importance as Spearman's proposal of his famous two-factor theory in 1904'. When Spearman tested people on various measures of cognitive abilities, he found that the correlations among the measures were almost always positive. People who scored high on one test tended to score high on the others. Spearman argued that performance on these tests was governed by one general characteristic, general intelligence factor. To account for the less perfect correlations between tests, Spearman proposed the existence of a task-specific factor.

Spearman's theory was based on an observation that various measures of performance or ability are positively correlated – a phenomenon termed positive manifold. Spearman explained this observation by arguing that all tests are influenced by this general factor, which he termed the psychometric g or just g. For example, if we administer three ability tests, say, Numerical Reasoning, Vocabulary and Mechanical Reasoning, we will invariably find that these measures are positively correlated. This correlation, Spearman would argue, is due to a more general factor, a general mental ability factor.

The intercorrelations among a set of tests can be represented as a matrix. Consider a correlation matrix reported by Spearman (1927: 147) in his famous book *The Abilities of Man*. In the table below we have the correlations among five tests, Mathematical judgment, Controlled association, Literary interpretation, Selective judgment and Spelling administered to 757 participants (the results are from Bosner, 1912, cited in Spearman, 1927).

	1	2	3	4	5
1 Mathematical judgment	—	0.485	0.400	0.397	0.295
2 Controlled association	0.485	—	0.397	0.397	0.247
3 Literary interpretation	0.400	0.397	—	0.335	0.275
4 Selective judgment	0.397	0.397	0.335	—	0.195
5 Spelling	0.295	0.247	0.275	0.195	—

Source: Spearman, 1927

Spearman made another very important observation about these correlations and other correlation matrices of this type. He noticed that, once the values in the matrix had been re-arranged, the size of the correlations tended to decrease as you moved from left to right in a row and from top to bottom as you moved down a column. For example, in the row for the test Spelling, the correlations go from 0.295 to 0.195 as you move from left to right along the row, and if you look at the column for Selective judgment you will see that the correlations decrease from 0.397 to 0.195. This pattern in the data led Spearman to postulate that there was an hierarchical ordering in the correlation matrix. He found that this pattern also showed that the tests varied in the amount of factor *g* they revealed. Correlations among tests to the left shared more of the factor *g* than tests to the right. In other words, a correlation matrix is hierarchically ordered if the size of the correlations decreases as you move from left to right in the correlation matrix and the correlations are all positive.

Spearman needed a way of demonstrating this concept of hierarchy mathematically. He noticed that if you partitioned the correlation matrix so that you looked at only four tests at a time, something interesting could be observed. He found that the difference of the products of the diagonal entries of the matrix tended to be 0 if the pattern in the overall matrix suggested an hierarchical ordering. He called this value the tetrad difference. Consider the following a partition of the correlation matrix presented earlier.

	Mathematical judgment	Literary interpretation
Selective judgment	0.397	0.335
Spelling	0.295	0.275

The tetrad difference is $(0.397 \times 0.275) - (0.335 \times 0.295) = 0.010$. Indeed most of the tetrads would be close to zero. Spearman had therefore found an empirical method (based on correlations) for determining if a correlation matrix was hierarchically ordered, and more importantly, a pattern of results that could be explained by his two-factor theory (Rogers, 1995).

Is There a Genetic Component to Intelligence? Did Burt clone the data? – data ain't always data!!

But is intelligence determined by the environment a person is reared in or is it determined by genetics? How do we study the degree to which heritability contributes to intelligence? This is one of the most important and contentious issues surrounding the study of human intelligence – the nature/nurture debate. Studies interested in the nature/nurture debate have often used twins, in particular identical twins reared apart, to discover influences of genetics and environment. Identical twins share the same genotype. If one were to find a substantial relationship between measures of intelligence of identical twins reared apart, then this would provide support for a genetic theory of intelligence.

The work of Sir Cyril Burt provided the most promise for resolving the nature/nurture debate. Burt's methodology was to examine identical twins reared apart, but also to compare the data obtained from these twins to other categories of paired children, such as identical twins reared together, non-identical twins reared together, siblings reared apart, siblings reared together, and unrelated children reared together. By using this methodology, the question of whether intelligence was genetically determined would be well and truly answered, or at least so Burt thought.

Burt and his co-workers tested numerous children in London. In 1943, Burt reported that the correlation on a measure of intelligence among a pair of 62 identical twins reared together was 0.86. He also reported a correlation of 0.771 based on the another sample of 15 identical twins. These results were exciting for the supporters of a genetic theory of intelligence. At last there was evidence supporting the theory. However, there was something fishy about the results being presented by Burt. Burt appeared to consistently report a correlation of 0.771 for identical twins reared apart. Moreover, there was amazing similarity in several of the correlations Burt was reporting. For example, in 1955, Burt reported that on a group test of intelligence for twins reared together, the correlation was 0.944; for identical twins reared apart the correlation was 0.771 and for unrelated children reared together the correlation was 0.281. Exactly the same correlations (to 3 decimal places!) were again reported in 1966. In addition, the 1955 study reported correlation of 0.490 and 0.563 for tests of reading and arithmetic respectively for siblings reared apart. The same correlation appeared in the 1996 study for the same group – the only difference was that the sample size had increased from 131 in 1955 to 151 in 1966!!

Burt's views on intelligence were controversial, but his data raised extra, more serious questions. Was this a case of scientific fraud or just a case of sloppiness? Kamin (1974) noted the remarkable consistency in Burt's results and questioned their veracity. Indeed, in 1976, Oliver Gillie, a medical reporter for the London *Times*, placed an ad in the paper asking if Margaret Howard or J. Conway could please contact him. Howard and Conway were research assistants who assisted Burt and their names appeared in some of the journal articles. No one replied. It was alleged that the two women did not exist and that Burt had made up the data to fit his genetic theories of intelligence. Abelson (1995: 102) argues that perhaps Burt was treated unfairly. Abelson noted:

> There is a benign explanation of the identity between early and late results, despite added cases. A reasonable conjecture is that not all of the measures were administered to the new cases. Because cases were hard to find, it is not unlikely that some compromises were made in the interest of fattening the total N. One such compromise might have been to omit some of the measures on some batches of cases. ... But this case makes the point that something that looks fishy might be okay (albeit poorly set forth by an author who did not make clear what was going on). Thus one should not be too quick to cry fraud.

Here then we have a case of detection where the statistical sleuth has looked at a set of results and found something fishy. In the Burt example, there was too much consistency in the results. In most of our research we look for replication of results. By replicating certain results we provide evidence for the validity of those results. But as students of statistics we are aware of the concept of variability. We may obtain similar results, but possibly not identical results (Rogers, 1995).

Are Social Factors More Important than Individual Inclinations? Durkheim's study on suicide (The use of secondary data)

Emile Durkheim held that social groups have a collective inclination for action, quite their own, and are the source of all individual inclinations, including suicidal actions (1897). He is the opposite of the statisticians cited above. Durkheim argued that biological, psychological and social psychological factors remain constant from one group to another or from one time to another.

Durkheim lived at the same time as Sherlock Holmes. Sociology was not taught as a discipline in Holmes's day. Durkheim was, therefore, one of the first theorists to try to define the discipline and to distinguish it from other disciplines such as philosophy and psychology.

Durkheim was a sleuth. He saw the incongruous. He noticed that phenomena like suicide were intensely personal. What more personal, and individual, an act could there be? Suicide appeared to be an intensely personal act that involved complex personal decision-making before a decision to die was made. A person's own psyche, own feelings, surely, dictated the course of action. Durkheim noticed, however, not only the *incidence* of suicide but *rates* of suicide. He saw patterns in the data that showed that suicides appeared to occur in the same proportions for different social groups over time. How could this be? Do different social groups, like doctors, set a quota of suicides each year?

Durkheim was a data collector and a creative problem-solver. His secondary data analysis drew on 26,000 cases of suicide that were classified separately by age, sex, marital status and the presence or absence of children. 'M. Mauss alone performed the heavy task' (1970: 39). The statistics were taken from official reports held by the Bureau of Legal Statistics, and other official and academic sources.

Let's start with Durkheim's conclusions before examining some of the data that he analysed:

> Victims of suicide are in an infinite minority, which is widely dispersed; each one of them performs his act separately, without knowing that others are doing the same; and yet, so long as society remains unchanged the number of suicides remains the same. Therefore, all these individual manifestations, however independent of one another they seem, must surely actually result from a single group of causes, which dominate individuals. Otherwise how could we explain that all these individual wills, ignorant of one another's existence, annually achieve the same end in the same numbers? At least for the most part they have no effect upon one another; they are in no way conjoined; yet everything takes place as if they were obeying a single order. There must then be some force in their common environment inclining them all in the same direction, whose greater or lesser strength causes the greater or less number of suicides. Now the effects revealing this force vary not according to organic and cosmic environments but solely according to the state of the social environment. This force must then be collective. In other words, each people has collectively an inclination of its own to suicide, on which the size of its contribution to voluntary death depends. (Durkheim, 1970: 304–5)

This short narrative is both a theoretical hypothesis and a conclusion in Durkheim's study. Figure 6.12 maps his 'cause and effect' statement.

Let's use Durkheim's examples from the statistics to show why he arrived at this theoretical model. When Durkheim summarized the suicide statistics by religion, for example in Table 6.18, he found that 'everywhere without exception, Protestants show far more suicides than the followers of other confessions' (1970: 154). The difference varied between a 20 to 30 per cent minimum and a maximum of 300 per cent. Jewish people committed suicide less than Catholics and Catholics less than Protestants. But why? Was the difference based on prohibition of suicide? No. Both Catholicism and

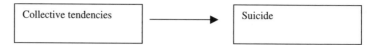

FIGURE 6.12   *Durkheim's theoretical hypothesis on suicide*

TABLE 6.18   *Suicides in different countries per million persons of each confession (adapted from Durkheim, 1952: 154)*

	Protestants	Catholics	Jews
Austria (1852–9)	79.5	51.3	20.7
Prussia (1849–55)	159.9	49.6	46.4
Prussia (1869–72)	187	69	96
Prussia (1890)	240	100	180
Baden (1852–62)	139	117	87
Baden (1870–4)	171	136.7	124
Baden (1878–88)	242	170	210
Bavaria (1844–56)	135.4	49.1	105.9
Bavaria (1884–91)	224	94	193
Wuttemberg (1846–60)	113.5	77.9	65.6
Wuttemberg (1873–6)	190	120	60
Wuttemberg (1881–90)	170	119	142

Protestantism penalized suicides 'with great severity' (1970: 157). What, then, made the difference? 'The only essential difference between Catholicism and Protestantism is that the second permits free inquiry to a far greater degree than the first' (1970: 157). 'Free inquiry', though, was for Durkheim only the effect of another cause. Catholicism has fewer common beliefs and practices than Protestantism. It has a creed, a set of beliefs, that tie the group together and there is therefore a greater the integration of the group: 'the greater the concessions a confessional group makes to individual judgement, the less it dominates lives, the less its cohesion and vitality' (1970: 159). Durkheim concluded, therefore, 'that the superiority of Protestantism with respect to suicide results from its being a less strongly integrated church than the Catholic Church' (1970: 159).

We can now break down Durkheim's more general theoretical hypothesis into a more specific hypothesis, represented in Figure 6.13. The higher the integration of a social group, the lower the suicide rate.

Durkheim extended this idea of integration to other statistics and other social groups. For example, from Tables 6.19 and 6.20, Durkheim concluded that 'it appears that marriage has indeed a preservative effect of its own against suicide' (1970: 198). Coefficient of preservation is the ratio of the suicide rates of two groups of the same age and sex. For example, if the suicide rate of unmarried men were 400 per million and that of married men of the same age only 100 per million, then the coefficient of preservation would be 3. The lower the suicide rate of a group, the higher its coefficient.

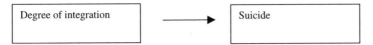

FIGURE 6.13   *Durkheim's hypothesis of degree of integration*

TABLE 6.19   *Influences of the family on suicide, unmarried men (adapted from Durkheim, 1970: 197–8)*

	Suicide rate	Coefficient of preservation in relation to unmarried men
Unmarried men 45 years old	975	. . .
Husbands with children	336	2.9
Husbands without children	644	1.5
Unmarried men 60 years old	1,504	. . .
Widowers with children	937	1.6
Widowers without children	1,258	1.2

TABLE 6.20   *Influences of the family on suicide, unmarried women (adapted from Durkheim, 1970: 197–8)*

	Suicide rate	Coefficient of preservation in relation to unmarried women
Unmarried women 42 years old	150	. . .
Wives with children	79	1.89
Wives without children	221	0.67
Unmarried women 60 years old	196	
Widows with children	186	1.06
Widows without children	322	0.60

For Durkheim, marriage and domestic society, like religious society, is a powerful counteragent against suicide.

Durkheim found something else happening with marriage statistics. The greater the number of divorces, the greater the number of suicides. He did not call this phenomenon 'disintegration', but an aspect of 'regulation'. The statistics on the relationship between divorce and suicide did not mean that there were more bad wives or husbands, but that the customs and laws surrounding marriage and divorce had changed. 'Divorce is never granted except out of respect for a pre-existing state of customs. If the public conscience had not gradually decided that the indissolubility of the conjugal bond is unreasonable, no legislator would never have thought of making it easier to break up' (1970: 273). When divorce takes a legal form it weakens the moral structures assisting integration. The law assists, does not restrain, suicide.

Durkheim created the construct **anomy** to describe the changes in 'regulation' and the weakening of social group norms. Figure 6.14 summarizes this second major hypothesis that relates to the idea of collective tendencies.

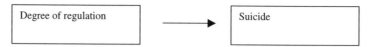

FIGURE 6.14   *Durkheim's hypothesis of degree of regulation*

Both integration and regulation contributed towards suicide and both make up the collective tendency. Durkheim labelled the different types of suicide according to the degree and overlap of integration or regulation. An unmarried person who committed suicide might be labelled an 'egoistic suicide', because that person no longer had his or her original basis for existence in life. A divorced person might be labelled an 'anomic suicide' because the social activity, marriage, lacked its original regulation. Durkheim also identified a third type of social cause of suicide – 'altruistic suicide' – where individuals are obliged to kill themselves. 'Celts were known who bound themselves to suffer death in consideration of wine or money' (1970: 222).

Altruistic suicide represents overly strong regulation of individuals; for example, the Hindu requirement that widows commit ritual suicide upon the funeral pyre. Where there is excessive regulation, the demands of society become so great that suicide varies directly rather than inversely with the degree of integration. Durkheim uses statistics from military suicides to show that the officer corps, because of the honour code, has higher suicides than lower ranks. The officer corps, highly integrated, should, one would suppose, have fewer suicides than other ranks.

Durkheim's category of 'altruistic suicide' shows us that he was acutely aware of the problems with different types of claims made by the 'individual' and by 'society'. His theories appear very conservative but in his private life he would, by modern standards, be defined as liberal.

Integration and regulation are 'functions' in Durkheim's work. They are real social causes that exist independently of a person's individual psychology. They form the basis of the 'collective tendencies' that deliver the proportion of suicides that we can observe in suicide rates. But these 'functions' affect more than one social act, like suicide. In Durkheim's theory they affect all society.

Durkheim, of course, did not escape criticism or critique. Like Sherlock Holmes, he was captured by the biases and prejudices of his day. 'Women's sexual needs,' says Durkheim, 'have less of a mental character because, generally speaking, her mental life is less developed' (1970: 272). Women have 'no great intellectual needs' (1970: 166). Such assumptions, one would assume, would affect Durkheim's perceptions about the constructs that he created. But the problem of 'definition' and 'constructs' goes further. The very records that Durkheim relied on can be problematic. Durkheim was not interested in the 'idiographic'. He did not investigate the definitions that individuals or groups involved might apply to the 'suicide act'. He did not interview relatives and friends caught up in the death – or the police and the courts. All these people or groups might affect what ended up being a 'suicide statistic'. 'It has been repeatedly pointed out by scientific students of the problem that suicide cannot be subject to statistical evaluation, since all too many suicides are not reported as such. Those who kill themselves through automobile accidents are almost never recorded as suicides; those who sustain serious injuries during an attempt to commit suicide and die weeks or months later of these injuries or of intercurrent infections are never registered as suicides; a great many genuine suicides are concealed by families; and suicidal attempts, no matter how serious, never find their way into the tables of vital statistics' (Zilboorg, cited in Durkheim, 1970: 18).

Durkheim's work, despite flaws, shows the benefits in using secondary data. There is a range of formal agencies in modern societies that collect data on topics ranging from suicide to number of cars in each household. There is also a range of studies, like Durkheim's, that can be revisited and mined – for critique or for extension.

SUMMARY

The good statistical sleuth does not treat statistical distributions as universal laws. 'We must hunt for cases', says the famous statistician, Karl Pearson (cited in Yule and Kendall, 1937: 186). Famous statistical measures were developed in response to an interest in fundamental issues surrounding human behaviour. Famous sociological theories were developed in response to interpretations of statistical evidence.

Quantitative research methods in social science research are often involved in the investigation of relationships between variables. The idea of correlation is central to this type of inquiry. The correlation coefficient provides a summary measure of the extent and direction of the relationship between two variables. This is a nomothetic approach to understanding association. But the origin of the correlation coefficient lies in the scatterplot which is idiographic in nature, plotting individual data points. Indeed the identification of outliers (individual data points that don't fit the trend!) is an important reason for constructing a scatterplot.

Correlation is closely related to prediction and statistical regression. Prediction is estimation. What regression allows us to do is to make an estimate that is better than simply an educated guess. Regression is a way of modelling data. Implicit in the idea of a model is error. Prediction, therefore, may not be precise. What the statistical sleuth tries to do is to get a model of the relationship between variables that best fits the data. The sleuth must remember that a linear model with just one explanatory variable is the simplest possible model and that care must be taken about any causal statements based on correlation models.

Correlation studies the relationship between variables. Inference allows the sleuth to generalize results from samples to populations – from the particular to the general. We considered one-sample tests for comparing whether a sample comes from a population with certain characteristics, as well as two-sample tests – tests that allow us to make statements about the population means based on sample evidence. These are nomothetic tests – making generalizations about averages, not individuals.

We also investigated non-parametric or distribution-free tests. These tests do not make assumptions about the distribution of the population parameter. Distribution-free tests are not used as often in the social sciences as they could be or should be. For example, Micceri (1989) wrote an influential paper in which he presented strong evidence that commonly measured variables (including achievement and personality) in psychology are not normally distributed. Yet traditional techniques continue to be used. One reason why traditional tests such the t-test are commonly used is that they are robust – they seem to be reasonably accurate even when distributional assumptions are violated. None the less, we are keen for the reader to explore the alternative methods, especially randomization tests. These tests are useful not only when distributional assumptions are violated but also when the assumption of random sampling has also been violated.

Quetelet, Galton, Pearson, Spearman, Burt and Durkheim are all examples of the application of statistics to specific problems. Sometimes the statistical sleuth ends up with good statistics that do not support the theory – this is a good, not a bad, outcome. Sometimes the statistical sleuth, like Durkheim, develops an interesting theory, but the collection and origin of the statistics themselves become an issue.

The Statistical Inquirer provides additional lessons on correlation and regression. Use these lessons to better understand both the formula and their application.

MAIN POINTS

- A scatterplot is a graphical representation of the relationship between two variables. We can use scatterplots to check for trends and patterns in the data, and in particular, linear trends.
- Correlation is a numerical summary of the extent and direction of the relationship between two variables. The correlation coefficient ranges from –1 to 1. A correlation of 1 indicates perfect positive linear correlation; a correlation of –1 indicates perfect negative linear correlation.
- A contingency table is a useful way of cross-tabulating frequencies from two categorical variables. The chi-square statistic is used to test for evidence of independence of two categorical variables.
- Statistical inference allows the researcher to generalize findings from samples to populations. The concept of a sampling distribution is important in statistical inference. We make decisions about the null hypothesis by determining whether the obtained statistic is relatively rare or common in the sampling distribution of that statistic.

- One-sample tests such as the z test and the one-sample t-test are used to test whether a sample is drawn from a population with certain parameter values. The chi-square test for goodness of fit allows comparison of actual frequencies with theoretical or expected frequencies.
- We can compare two independent samples and make conclusions about their respective parent populations using the t-test for independent samples. The Mann-Whitney U test is a distribution-free alternative to the independent samples t-test.
- If samples are related or matched then the related samples t-test allows us to test whether the population means are equal or not. The Wilcoxon signed rank test is the distribution-free analogue of the related samples test.
- The independence of two categorical variables can be tested using the chi-square test.
- Randomization tests are useful alternatives to traditional statistical tests when distributional assumptions and random sampling assumptions have been violated.

REVIEW EXERCISES

1 A psychology department decides to evaluate the performance of its lecturers. Each lecturer teaches one subject. The department measures each lecturer on (1) the average grade for students completing the subject on a scale of 0 to 10, and (2) a measure of overall quality of lecture presentation on a scale from 0 to 5 (low scores indicating poor quality). The data are collected from 10 lecturers and presented below.

Mean grade	Mean quality rating
9.8	4.5
8.0	4.0
4.4	3.0
6.4	3.5
5.1	2.0
6.8	3.0
5.7	1.5
5.0	3.5
8.0	4.0
7.5	6.0

(a) Plot the relationship between mean quality of lecture rating and mean grade scores. How would you describe this relationship?

(b) Compute the correlation coefficient for quality of lectures and grade score. Interpret the correlation coefficient.

(c) Using quality to predict grade scores, find the equation of the form $Y = a + bX$ which makes the best prediction.

(d) What is your best estimate of the expected mean grade when the quality rating of lecturers is 2.5?

2 Explain in your own words what is meant by the standard error of the estimate of Y.

3 In a study linking criminality and identical versus fraternal twins, 15 identical-twin pairs and 17 fraternal-twin pairs were studied. It was found that of the 15 identical-twin pairs, 10 pairs had two criminals while the remaining pairs had one criminal. Of the 17 fraternal-twin pairs, five pairs had two criminals, while the remaining pairs had one criminal. Construct a contingency table for these data. Test whether the two variables are independent using a chi-square test. (Based on Guilford, 1965.)

4 A media lecturer is interested in the impact of viewing a Woody Allen comedy on the mood of the viewers. He hypothesizes that the mood of the viewers will be different after viewing the film. He uses the measure of mood on which high scores indicate positive mood. The score of the 10 participating viewers are recorded below:

Before: 12 16 17 10 18 16 15 11 12 15
After: 15 16 17 13 16 17 16 13 13 16

What statistical test would you use to test the researcher's hypothesis? Perform the test and interpret the results.

5 You will need to carry out this exercise with the assistance of your teacher and some very obliging colleagues. For each of 10 fellow students, measure their head circumference in centimetres (or inches) and the length of their foot (in cm or inches). Use SPSS or Excel to find the correlation between head circumference and length of foot. Interpret your findings.

6 Use the Rawstorne's computer anxiety data to find whether males and females differ on the variable 'confid1' – confidence using computers. High scores on this variable mean greater confidence. State which test you would use and why. Use SPSS or Excel to conduct the analysis.

7 Ask 10 of your fellow male students and 10 of your fellow female students whether they prefer rock, jazz or classical music. They must choose only one category. Construct the contingency table. Are the two variables related or independent?

REFERENCES

Abelson, R.P. (1995) *Statistics as Principled Argument.* Hillsdale, NJ: Lawrence Erlbaum Associates.

Agrest, A (1990) *Categorical Data Analysis.* New York: Wiley.

Baller, W.R. (1936) 'A study of the present states of adults who were mentally deficient', *Genetic Psychology Monography* 18: 165–244.

Bishop, Y.M.M, Fienberg, S.E. and Holland, P.W. (1975) *Discrete Multivarite Analysis.* Cambridge, MA: The MIT Press.

Burt, C. (1955) 'The evidence for the concept of intelligence', *British Journal of Educational Psychology,* 25: 158–77.

Burt, C. (1966). 'The genetic determination of differences in intelligence: a study of monozygotic twins reared together and apart', *British Journal of Psychology,* 57: 137–53.

Cohen, J. and Cohen P. (1983) *Applied Multiple Regression and Correlation Analysis for the Behavioural Sciences.* Hillsdale, NJ: Lawrence Erlbaum Associates.

Draper, N.R. and Smith, H. (1981) *Applied Regression Analysis.* New York: John Wiley and Sons.

Durkheim, E. (1964) *The Rules of Sociological Methods.* New York: Free Press.

Durkheim, E. (1970) *Suicide: a study in sociology.* London: Routledge and Kegan Paul.

Edgington, E.S. (1964) 'Randomization tests', *Journal of Psychology,* 57: 445–9.

Edgington, E.S. (1995) *Randomization Tests.* New York: Marcel Dekker.

Ferguson, G.A. (1959) *Statistical Analysis in Psychology and Education.* New York: McGraw-Hill.

Guilford, J.P. (1954) *Psychometric Methods.* New York: McGraw-Hill.

Guilford, J.P. (1965) *Fundamental Statistics in Psychology and Education.* New York: McGraw-Hill.

Hankins, F.H. (1968) *Adolphe Quetelet as Statistician.* New York: AMS Press.

Hayes, A.F. (1988) 'SPSS procedures for randomization tests', Behavior Research, Methods', *Instruments and Computers,* 30(3): 536–43.

Howell, D.C. (1992) *Statistical Methods for Psychology.* Belmont CA: Duxbury.

Innes, J.M. (1965) 'A case study of problem solving', *Bulletin of the British Psychological Society,* 18(61): 11–15.

Kamin, L. (1974) *The Science and Politics of IQ.* Hillsdale NJ: Erlbaum.

Kerlinger, F.N. and Pedhazur, E.J. (1973) *Multiple Regression in Behavioral Research.* New York: Holt, Rinehart and Winston.

May, R.B. and Hunter, M. (1993) 'Some advantages of permutation tests', *Canadian Psychology,* 34: 401–7.

Manly, B.F.J. (1991) *Randomization and Monte Carlo Methods in Biology.* London: Chapman and Hall.

Micceri, T. (1989) 'The unicorn, the normal curve, and other improbable creatures', *Psychological Bulletin,* 105: 156–66.

Moore, D.S. and McCabe, G.P. (1993) *Introduction to the Practice of Statistics.* New York: Freeman.

Spearman, C. (1927/1932) *The Abilities of Man.* London: Macmillan.

Queen, E. (1983) *The Dutch Shoe Mystery.* London: Hamlyn.

US Surgeon General (1964) Smoking and health. *Report to the Advisory Committee to the Surgeon General of the Public Health Service.* Washington, DC: US Government Printing Office.

Yule, G.U. and Kendall, M.G. (1937) *An Introduction to the Theory of Statistics.* London: Charles Griffin.

7
Summarizing and Presenting Results

'Quite so!'

'You see, Lady Swaffham, if ever you want to commit a murder, the thing you've got to do is to prevent people from associatin' their ideas. Most people don't associate anythin' – their ideas just roll about like so many dry peas on a tray, makin' a lot of noise an' goin' nowhere, but once you begin lettin' 'em string their peas into a necklace, it's goin' to be strong enough to hang you, what?'

'Dear me!' said Mrs Tommy Frayle, with a little scream, 'what a blessing it is none of my friends have any ideas at all!'

'Y'see,' said Lord Peter, balancing a piece of duck on his fork and frowning, 'it's only in Sherlock Holmes and stories like that, that people think things out logically. Or'nar'ly, if somebody tells you somethin' out of the way, you just say, 'By Jove!' or 'How sad!' an' leave it at that, an' half the time you forget about it, 'nless somethin' turns up afterwards to drive it home.' (Sayers, 1989: 118)

Lord Peter Wimsey
Whose Body?

Associatin' ideas is what quantitative research is about. Good research design and good data analysis assist in the process of associating ideas and coming to a conclusion. But we are not ended there. Research also has to be presented to readers – to an audience. Those readers and that audience have to be able to understand your research. Often research is not only for the immediate experts in your field but for a broader public, including policy makers and managers. If they cannot understand your work, and make the associations that you expect, then your good design and good analysis will be wasted.

The theme of this book has been detection and reasoning about evidence. The different styles of reasoning about evidence in detective fiction – deduction, induction, abduction – have their counterpart in social science and in statistics. But detectives like Sherlock Holmes sometimes mistake their guesses for deductions. Holmes 'meta-bets' – he constructs scenarios about real-world events that may or may not match up with those events. Detectives bet by meta-abduction, social scientists also test their abductions.

Inspector Wexford was not impressed by Sherlock Holmes's methods, as Burden recalls in *Simisola*:

Burden thought of something Wexford had once said to him about Sherlock Holmes, how you couldn't solve much by his methods. A pair of slippers with singed soles no more showed that their wearer had been suffering from a severe chill than that he had merely had cold feet. Nor could you deduce from a man's staring at a portrait on the wall that he was dwelling on the life and career of that portrait's subject, for he might equally be thinking of how it resembled his brother-in-law or was badly painted or needed cleaning. With human nature you could only guess – and try to guess right. (Rendell, 1994: 130)

Traditional ideas about 'deduction' raise traditional debates about 'laws' in social science. Holmes, for example, assumes that from a small set of facts he can deduce the whole chain of events, because he believes that events exist in law-like causal chains: 'all life is a great chain, the nature of which is known whenever we are shown a single link' (*Study in Scarlet*). This 'great chain', however, may be closer to the idea of **order at all points**, introduced in Chapter 1, rather than sets of laws to which we can refer our evidence. The great chain of society and culture – order at all points – is created by people and not by immutable unchangeable universal laws that govern society and culture.

Qualitative and quantitative research exist on a continuum. Ql and Qt researchers exist on a continuum and not as strict alternatives. Ql-oriented researchers will often find themselves needing to use statistical models and their ensuing graphic representations or software analysis programs that allow representation of data in categorical form. Qt-oriented researchers will find that they *cannot help but preserve* in their results the cultural order that the statistics attempt to measure.

The case studies that we have presented in the previous chapters are all examples of the qualitative and quantitative continuum. Hoftstede's research on intercultural communication variables like individualism, uncertainty avoidance, masculinity and power distance was deductive and nomothetic. Hofstede acknowledged the idiographic when he took into account the use of constructs in everyday life. He tried to to find observable phenomena from which the constructs of everyday life can be inferred (1984: 17).

Lazarsfeld's longitudinal study of the attitudes and behaviour of a panel of voters during a United States presidential campaign, in contrast, was inductive and nomothetic. He and his colleagues knew what they wanted to study, but they did not have a highly structured theoretical approach that determined the operationalization of their variables. In both cases, Hoftstede's and Lazarsfeld's, however, care was taken with **frame of reference** – the cultural and language contexts to which operational definitions, and questions, apply. Lazarsfeld's early triangulation of methods, his combining of the qualitative and the quantitative is a good example of an attempt at methods level to deal with order at all points:

1   Any phenomenon should be measured with objective observations as well as with introspective reports.
2   Case studies should be combined with statistical information.
3   Data gathering should be combined with information about the history of what is being studied.

4 Data from unobtrusive studies (e.g. observation) should be combined with questionnaire and other self-reported data. (cited Rogers, 1994: 285)

Methodologies can be deductive and inductive in quantitative research. Deduction, as a style of reasoning, certainly occurs in social science. But, like induction and abduction, it is closer to the 'probable' and 'possible' rather than the 'necessary', and if it is the 'necessary' then it is closer to C.S. Peirce's examples presented in Chapter 3 than it is to traditional science:

> I once landed at a seaport in a Turkish province; and as I was walking up to the house which I was to visit, I met a man upon horseback, surrounded by four horsemen holding a canopy over his head. As the governor of the province was the only personage I could think of who would be so greatly honored, I inferred that this was he. This was an hypothesis. (cited in Eco, 1983: 219)

This is a case of inferences based on conventions, not laws. All the case studies that we have presented to you raise the problem of methodology, hypothesis, research questions, identification and operationalization of constructs, measurement and judgements – inferences – about the results. The research designs themselves can be deductive – like those of Hofstede, or inductive – like those of Lazarsfeld. In the former, the research design has formalized hypotheses that are to be tested – there is less room for exploration. In the latter research design, there are research questions and more room for exploration. There can also be different degrees of nomotheticity in different research designs. The big 'nomothetic' studies seek answers to the very big picture, such as *Accounting for Tastes* (1999), presented in Chapter 5, which sought to answer questions about the relationship between social class and culture and did so by quantifying social class and relating it to cultural preferences.

It might be argued that we have not presented research examples that used abduction, or guessing. However, not surprisingly, there is an element of guessing in the whole process of a research project. Indeed, abduction is involved in the very *formation* of a hypothesis as 'an act of insight', the 'abductive suggestion' coming to us 'like a flash' (cited in Sebeok and Umiker-Sebeok, 1983: 18). Abduction is often the first step of social scientific reasoning.

The idea of 'guessing' and the idea of 'mistake' also go hand in hand. A guess can be wrong. A good research design and good data analysis reduce the chances of bias and error. As we have seen, bias and error can happen in many ways. They can happen with the styles of reasoning themselves, for example mistaking ideology for deduction (as in the case of Carl Jung). Error and bias can also happen in the operational definitions of constructs, the choice of measurement techniques, sampling, the wording of questions, the administration of the data-collecting instrument, data analysis and in the interpretation of results. A good social scientist, therefore, needs to be both a detective and a statistical sleuth (data snooper).

Openness and accountability and following the professional code of ethics are intended as good protections against acceptance of assertions and appeals to authority without presentation and testing of evidence. Other researchers should be able to test your methodology and critique your conclusions. Holmes and Lord Peter Wimsey continually berated the police for poor methodology. They argued that, in comparison to the police, they were not only exceptionally gifted individuals, but good methodologists – 'You know my method. It is founded upon the observation of trifles', says Holmes (*The Boscombe Valley Mystery*).

Professional codes of ethics are provided by the professional associations of the different disciplines of social science. The codes are sometimes made available on the internet site of the association. For instance, Appendix II is an example from the British Sociological Association internet site. The British and American Psychological Societies and other professional research groups outline their professional and ethics codes.

REPORTING EMPIRICAL RESEARCH

Detectives in detective fiction sometimes write reports. Many of them, of course, are not statistical in nature, although they are deductive. Ellery Queen, for example, often presents to the reader what he has written in his notebook. Chief Inspector Maigret, the French inspector, also writes down what he knows and what he plans to do:

1. Telegraph Rouen
2. Telegraph Niel's
3. Look at yard
4. Get information on Saint-Hilaire property
5. Finger-prints on knife
6. List of hotel visitors
7. Engineer's family Hotel du Commerce
8. People who left Sancerre Sunday the 26th
9. Announce reward, by town-crier, to anyone who met Gallet Saturday the 25th. (Simeon, 1977: 23)

Keeping a record of observations, of course, is essential to detection. The accumulation of evidence assists with the associatin' of ideas. The detective's final report is the narrative explaining what happened and who killed whom. In the case of *Maigret Stonewalled*, Maigret finds that the person assumed to have been murdered in fact committed suicide. The suicide had fabricated his death to look like a murder. Maigret does not report his findings to his superiors or the insurance company because of the tragic circumstances surrounding the death and the possible consequence if he released his findings. There was, therefore, an ethics element to what he did with his findings. Was Maigret right? Read the story.

The case studies presented in this book are good examples of reporting social scientific empirical research. There is a presentation of the problem, a literature review, methodology, findings and a conclusion. The journal articles that you will have read during the course of the review exercises in this book also give you a good indication of the standard formats for reporting quantitative research findings.

Table 2.3 provided an overview of the types of content that are addressed in both the design and reporting of quantitative research. But this overview is not complete. Most articles in social science journals begin with an ABSTRACT, set off from the text of the article. An abstract is a summary of the research findings and is normally about 150 words in length. The abstract gives an overview of the purpose of the research, the methods, results and conclusions. Many of the database searches in modern university libraries are not full-text, but searches of words in abstracts.

The first section of an article is the INTRODUCTION. The introduction may not appear as a heading, but it tells the reader the rationale for the research, background to the research (previous studies) and normally ends in a formal statement(s) of hypothesis(es). Some articles have sub-headings such as BACKGROUND and LITERATURE REVIEW. As we saw in Chapter 2 in the review of the studies in the sociology of journalism, a literature review is not simply a rote recitation of what people said – parrot fashion – but an evaluation and a synthesis of previous studies.

The METHOD section gives the reader the specific rules for replicating your study. It contains detailed information about how the study was conducted. It tells the reader who the **participants** or subjects of the study were, the **procedures** (a common sub-heading) that were used to conduct the study, how variables were operationally defined, and which **measures** were used (a common sub-heading).

The RESULTS section provides readers with a summary of the findings of the research. It is here that the main findings relevant to the hypothesis or hypotheses are presented and, in some cases, additional information as well. It is in the results that the reader will encounter the relevant statistical notation, tables and graphs. Table 7.1, taken from *Accounting for Tastes*,

TABLE 7.1   *Example from Accounting for Tastes: combined music genre preferences by gender*

Genres with no gender differences	'Female' genres	'Male' genres
Classical	Light classical ***	Heavy metal***
Avant-garde	Musicals***	Rock**
Traditional jazz	Religious***	Blues**
Modern jazz	Easy listening***	Alternative rock**
Big band	Top 40**	Folk**
	Soul*	Techno**
	Opera*	Country and Western*

* p $<$ 0.1; ** p $<$ 0.001; *** p $<$ 0.0001.

discussed in Chapter 5, is an example of tabular results and notation. The table is derived from the combined preferences for music types and shows those music genres for which there is no difference between males and females in their musical preferences and those that are more likely to be favoured by either males or females.

Notice that the p-value is stated clearly and simply at the bottom of the table, although in this case the chi-square values and degrees of freedom are not shown (indeed the type of statistic used is not stated in the text). The data, though, is clearly categorical in nature.

Many of the statistics in the reporting of empirical results are presented as p-values. If you are reading research results and there is no background statistic, then it is best to ignore the values for statistics such as t, r, chi-square, and so on, and look for p. If you are writing the research, then it is useful to provide the background statistic for the reader's information.

In Table 7.1 the p-values have an asterisk. This shows that the associations are significant. If the p-value is less than 0.01, it means that the probability of the result occurring by chance is less than 10 per cent (behavioural research often sets the minimum at 0.05, less than 5 per cent). If the p-value is less than 0.001, then the probability of the result occurring by chance is less than one-tenth of 1 per cent, and so on.

The results section of a report sometimes combines description of results and detailed analysis, as in the case of *Accounting for Tastes*. However, detailed analysis is often left for a separate DISCUSSION section. The discussion section presents the implications of the research and the extent to which the hypotheses of the research were supported by the data. Indeed, the author evaluates alternative explanations for the data and limitations that might have been imposed or the study or problems that might have emerged.

A CONCLUSION or SUMMARY, like the abstract, brings together for the reader all the strands of the report. It includes all the significant information about methods, findings and discussion.

Writing Style, Narrative Style

A report, essay, article or thesis describing the empirical results of a research study requires a writing style, a narrative skill, which achieves a high level of readability. You will find conventions and strategies for writing in a range of resources (Anderson and Poole, 1994; Peters, 1985).

As a rule of thumb: (1) avoid colloquial, conversational and subjective modes of expression and (2) avoid abbreviations such as & and don't. 'Scientific writing is not of a personal or conversational nature and for this reason the third person is commonly used. As a general rule, personal pronouns such as I, we, you, me, my, our and us should not appear, except in quotations' (Anderson and Poole, 1994: 6).

The 'third person' rule holds in most cases. But sometimes the narrative style may require the more personal touch. Social science projects, for example, may use a methodology that requires the researcher to report their own subjective experiences – especially where they have been participant observers.

Good research work can be marred by bad reporting; 'proper presentation is an integral part of the whole project' (Anderson and Poole, 1994: 6). You will, no doubt, develop your own style for reporting results and arguing your case. But, whatever your style, your presentation should ensure that:

1 people will understand and accept the evidence in the form you have provided it;
2 the evidence is instrumental in making the case or in supporting the claim;
3 the evidence is at an appropriate technical and intellectual level for the proposed readers;
4 the readers know and respect the sources of evidence.

Detection and Deception

The problems you face in developing a narrative for your results are in many ways no different from those faced by detectives in detective fiction. You have to show that you understand your methods and that your reasoning about your results is sound. Detectives need tools, methods, to collect their data. They are creative problem-solvers who know that it is important to understand the reasoning behind their methods. Detectives make judgements about individual pieces of evidence that may or may not be signs of what really happened. Holmes and Lord Peter Wimsey were angry with police detectives precisely because they believed that the police methods did not yield real signs, real clues.

A social scientist often has to be a good detective and a good statistical sleuth. Social scientists confront the general and the particular, the macro and the micro, in theory and in practice. For example, theoreticians like Durkheim used rates of suicide, a general classification, to show how society regulates and integrates its members. In doing so he lost information, especially information about the circumstances that underpinned the classification of the 'suicide' act itself.

But even when we are confident that our constructs measure what we say they measure, we have to be careful with the statistical measures that we choose. There are, as you have seen, quite complex statistical measures for interpreting and summarizing individual scores, or values, that are obtained from a study. Equations have definition, like any other construct, and need to be carefully understood before they are used. They are general classifications that can either enhance or obscure the real meaning of the data that you are analysing.

This text is only an introduction to methods and basic statistics. Some of the theory and methods look and are complex. Some of the statistics are complex. But, as Sherlock Holmes says, 'Come, the game is afoot!'

REFERENCES

Anderson, J. and Poole, M. (1994) *Thesis and Assignment Writing*. Brisbane: John Wiley and Sons.

Bennett, T., Emmison, M. and Frow, J. (1999) *Accounting for Tastes: Australian Everyday Culture*. Cambridge: Cambridge University Press.

Doyle, Arthur Conan (1952) *The Complete Sherlock Holmes*. Garden City, New York: Doubleday.

Eco, U. (1983) 'Horns, hooves, insteps', in U. Eco and T. Sebeok (eds), *The Sign of Three: Dupin, Holmes, Pierce*. Bloomington, IN: Indiana University Press.

Hofstede, G. (1984) *Culture's Consequences: International differences in work-related values*. Beverley Hills, CA: Sage.

Peters, P. (1985) *Strategies for Student Writers*. Brisbane: John Wiley and Sons.

Rendell, R. (1994) *Simisola*. London: Random House.

Rogers, E.M. (1994) *A History of Communication Study*. New York: Free Press.

Sayers, D. (1989) *Whose Body?* Sevenoaks: New English Library.

Sebeok, T.A. and Umiker-Sebeok, J. (1983) 'You know my method', in U. Eco and T. Sebeok (eds), *The Sign of Three: Dupin, Holmes, Pierce*. Bloomington, IN: Indiana University Press.

Simeon, G. (1977) *Maigret Stonewalled*. Harmondsworth: Penguin.

Appendix I

Sample Letter for Informed Consent

School/Division Title   Murdoch University logo as per standard
                                         letterhead

Project Title: Adult Literacy in Australia.

I am a (PhD/Honours/fourth year Psychology) student (member of staff) at Murdoch University investigating the level of literacy among adults in Australia. The purpose of this study is to find out what causes low levels of literacy among some adults in Australia and to investigate how levels of literacy in Australia can be improved.

You can help in this study by consenting to complete a survey. The time to complete the survey will vary, however, it is anticipated that no more than two hours will be necessary. Contained in the survey are questions about level of education, income, and other questions which may be seen as personal and private. Therefore, participants can decide to withdraw their consent at any time. All information given during the survey is confidential and no names or other information which might identify you will be used in any publication arising from the research.

If you are willing to participate in this study, could you please complete the details below. If you have any questions about this project please feel free to contact either myself (investigator's name), on 9234 5678 or my supervisor, Dr John Smith, on 9360 2345.

My supervisor and I are happy to discuss with you any concerns you may have on how this study has been conducted, or alternatively you can contact Murdoch University's Human Research Ethics Committee on 9360 6677.

****

I (the participant) have read the information above. Any questions I have asked have been answered to my satisfaction. I agree to take part in this activity, however, I know that I may change my mind and stop at any time (where applicable add – without prejudice to my future medical treatment).

I understand that all information provided is treated as confidential and will not be released by the investigator unless required to do so by law.

I agree that research data gathered for this study may be published provided my name or other information which might identify me is not used.

Participant/Authorised Representative:

Date:

Investigator:

Date:

Investigator's Name:

Appendix II

BSA Statement of Ethical Practice

The British Sociological Association gratefully acknowledges the use made of the ethical codes produced by the American Sociological Association, the Association of Social Anthropologists of the Commonwealth and the Social Research Association.

Styles of sociological work are diverse and subject to change, not least because sociologists work within a wide variety of settings. Sociologists, in carrying out their work, inevitably face ethical, and sometimes legal, dilemmas which arise out of competing obligations and conflicts of interest. The following statement aims to alert the members of the Association to issues that raise ethical concerns and to indicate potential problems and conflicts of interest that might arise in the course of their professional activities.

While they are not exhaustive, the statement points to a set of obligations to which members should normally adhere as principles for guiding their conduct. Departures from the principles should be the result of deliberation and not ignorance. The strength of this statement and its binding force rest ultimately on active discussion, reflection, and continued use by sociologists. In addition, the statement will help to communicate the professional position of sociologists to others, especially those involved in or affected by the activities of sociologists.

The statement is meant, primarily, to inform members' ethical judgements rather than to impose on them an external set of standards. The purpose is to make members aware of the ethical issues that may arise in their work, and to encourage them to educate themselves and their colleagues to behave ethically. The statement does not, therefore, provide a set of recipes for resolving ethical choices or dilemmas, but recognises that often it will be necessary to make such choices on the basis of principles and values, and the (often conflicting) interests of those involved.

PROFESSIONAL INTEGRITY

Members should strive to maintain the integrity of sociological enquiry as a discipline, the freedom to research and study, and to publish and promote the results of sociological research. Members have a responsibility both to safeguard the proper interests of those involved in or affected by their work, and to report their findings accurately and truthfully. They need to consider the effects of their involvements and the consequences of their work or its misuse for those they study and other interested parties.

While recognising that training and skill are necessary to the conduct of social research, members should themselves recognise the boundaries of their professional competence. They should not accept work of a kind that they are not qualified to carry out. Members should satisfy themselves that the research they undertake is worthwhile and that the techniques proposed are appropriate. They should be clear about the limits of their detachment from and involvement in their areas of study.

Members should be careful not to claim an expertise in areas outside those that would be recognised academically as their true fields of expertise. Particularly in their relations with the media, members should have regard for the reputation of the discipline and refrain from offering expert commentaries in a form that would appear to give credence to material which, as researchers, they would regard as comprising inadequate or tendentious evidence.

RELATIONS WITH AND RESPONSIBILITIES TOWARDS RESEARCH PARTICIPANTS

Sociologists, when they carry out research, enter into personal and moral relationships with those they study, be they individuals, households, social groups or corporate entities. Although sociologists, like other researchers are committed to the advancement of knowledge, that goal does not, of itself, provide an entitlement to override the rights of others. Members must satisfy themselves that a study is necessary for the furtherance of knowledge before embarking upon it. Members should be aware that they have some responsibility for the use to which their research may be put. Discharging that responsibility may on occasion be difficult, especially in situations of social conflict, competing social interests or where there is unanticipated misuse of the research by third parties.

1. Relationships with research participants
   - Sociologists have a responsibility to ensure that the physical, social and psychological well-being of research participants is not adversely affected by the research. They should strive to protect the rights of those they study, their interests, sensitivities and privacy, while recognising the difficulty of balancing potentially conflicting interests. Because sociologists study the relatively powerless as well as those more powerful than themselves, research relationships are frequently characterised by disparities of power and status. Despite this, research relationships should be characterised, whenever possible, by trust. In some cases, where the public interest dictates otherwise and particularly where power is being abused, obligations of trust and protection may weigh less heavily. Nevertheless, these obligations should not be discarded lightly.
   - As far as possible sociological research should be based on the freely given informed consent of those studied. This implies a responsibility on the sociologist to explain as fully as possible, and in terms meaningful to participants, what the research is about, who is undertaking and financing it, why it is being undertaken, and how it is to be promoted.
     - (i) Research participants should be made aware of their right to refuse participation whenever and for whatever reason they wish.
     - (ii) Research participants should understand how far they will be afforded anonymity and confidentiality and should be able to reject the use of data-gathering devices such as tape recorders and video cameras. Sociologists should be careful, on the one hand, not to give

unrealistic guarantees of confidentiality and, on the other, not to permit communication of research films or records to audiences other than those to which the research participants have agreed.

- (iii) Where there is a likelihood that data may be shared with other researchers, the potential uses to which the data might be put may need to be discussed with research participants.
- (iv) When making notes, filming or recording for research purposes, sociologists should make clear to research participants the purpose of the notes, filming or recording, and, as precisely as possible, to whom it will be communicated.
- (v) It should also be borne in mind that in some research contexts, especially those involving field research, it may be necessary for the obtaining of consent to be regarded, not as a once-and-for-all prior event, but as a process, subject to renegotiation over time. In addition, particular care may need to be taken during periods of prolonged field-work where it is easy for research participants to forget that they are being studied.
- (vi) In some situations access to a research setting is gained via a 'gate-keeper'. In these situations members should adhere to the principle of obtaining informed consent directly from the research participants to whom access is required, while at the same time taking account of the gatekeeper's interest. Since the relationship between the research participant and the gatekeeper may continue long after the sociologist has left the research setting, care should be taken not to disturb that relationship unduly.
- It is incumbent upon members to be aware of the possible consequences of their work. Wherever possible they should attempt to anticipate, and to guard against, consequences for research participants which can be pre-dicted to be harmful. Members are not absolved from this responsibility by the consent given by research participants.
- In many of its guises, social research intrudes into the lives of those studied. While some participants in sociological research may find the experience a positive and welcome one, for others, the experience may be disturbing. Even if not exposed to harm, those studied may feel wronged by aspects of the research process. This can be particularly so if they perceive apparent intrusions into their private and personal worlds, or where research gives rise to false hopes, uncalled for self-knowledge, or unnecessary anxiety. Members should consider carefully the possibility that the research experi-ence may be a disturbing one and, normally, should attempt to minimise disturbance to those participating in research. It should be borne in mind that decisions made on the basis of research may have effects on individuals as members of a group, even if individual research participants are pro-tected by confidentiality and anonymity.
- Special care should be taken where research participants are particularly vulnerable by virtue of factors such as age, social status and powerlessness. Where research participants are ill or too young or too old to participate, proxies may need to be used in order to gather data. In these situations care should be taken not to intrude on the personal space of the person to whom the data ultimately refer, or to disturb the relationship between this person and the proxy. Where it can be inferred that the person about whom data

are sought would object to supplying certain kinds of information, that material should not be sought from the proxy.

2. Covert research

There are serious ethical dangers in the use of covert research but covert methods may avoid certain problems. For instance, difficulties arise when research participants change their behaviour because they know they are being studied. Researchers may also face problems when access to spheres of social life is closed to social scientists by powerful or secretive interests. However, covert methods violate the principles of informed consent and may invade the privacy of those being studied. Participant or non-participant observation in non-public spaces or experimental manipulation of research participants without their knowledge should be resorted to only where it is impossible to use other methods to obtain essential data. In such studies it is important to safeguard the anonymity of research participants. Ideally, where informed consent has not been obtained prior to the research it should be obtained post-hoc.

3. Anonymity, privacy and confidentiality
   1. The anonymity and privacy of those who participate in the research process should be respected. Personal information concerning research participants should be kept confidential. In some cases it may be necessary to decide whether it is proper or appropriate even to record certain kinds of sensitive information.
   2. Where possible, threats to the confidentiality and anonymity of research data should be anticipated by researchers. The identities and research records of those participating in research should be kept confidential whether or not an explicit pledge of confidentiality has been given. Appropriate measures should be taken to store research data in a secure manner. Members should have regard to their obligations under the Data Protection Act. Where appropriate and practicable, methods for preserving the privacy of data should be used. These may include the removal of identifiers, the use of pseudonyms and other technical means for breaking the link between data and identifiable individuals such as 'broadbanding' or micro-aggregation. Members should also take care to prevent data being published or released in a form which would permit the actual or potential identification of research participants. Potential informants and research participants, especially those possessing a combination of attributes which make them readily identifiable, may need to be reminded that it can be difficult to disguise their identity without introducing an unacceptably large measure of distortion into the data.
   3. Guarantees of confidentiality and anonymity given to research participants must be honoured, unless there are clear and overriding reasons to do otherwise. Other people, such as colleagues, research staff or others, given access to the data must also be made aware of their obligations in this respect. By the same token, sociologists should respect the efforts taken by other researchers to maintain anonymity. Research data given in confidence do not enjoy legal privilege, that is they may be liable to subpoena by a court. Research participants may also need to be made aware that it may not be possible to avoid legal threats to the privacy of the data.

4. There may be less compelling grounds for extending guarantees of privacy or confidentiality to public organisations, collectivities, governments, officials or agencies than to individuals or small groups. Nevertheless, where guarantees have been given they should be honoured, unless there are clear and compelling reasons not to do so.

4. Reputation of the Discipline
During their research members should avoid, where they can, actions which may have deleterious consequences for sociologists who come after them or which might undermine the reputation of sociology as a discipline.

RELATIONS WITH AND RESPONSIBILITIES TOWARDS SPONSORS AND/OR FUNDERS

A common interest exists between sponsor, funder and sociologist as long as the aim of the social inquiry is to advance knowledge, although such knowledge may only be of limited benefit to the sponsor and the funder. That relationship is best served if the atmosphere is conducive to high professional standards. Members should attempt to ensure that sponsors and/or funders appreciate the obligations that sociologists have not only to them, but also to society at large, research participants and professional colleagues and the sociological community. The relationship between sponsors or funders and social researchers should be such as to enable social inquiry to be undertaken as objectively as possible. Research should be undertaken with a view to providing information or explanation rather than being constrained to reach particular conclusions or prescribe particular courses of action.

1. Clarifying obligations, roles and rights
   - Members should clarify in advance the respective obligations of funders and researchers where possible in the form of a written contract. They should refer the sponsor or funder to the relevant parts of the professional code to which they adhere. Members should also be careful not to promise or imply acceptance of conditions which are contrary to their professional ethics or competing commitments. Where some or all of those involved in the research are also acting as sponsors and/or funders of research the potential for conflict between the different roles and interests should also be made clear to them.
   - Members should also recognise their own general or specific obligations to the sponsors whether contractually defined or only the subject of informal and often unwritten agreements. They should be honest and candid about their qualifications and expertise, the limitations, advantages and disadvantages of the various methods of analysis and data, and acknowledge the necessity for discretion with confidential information obtained from sponsors. They should also try not to conceal factors which are likely to affect satisfactory conditions or the completion of a proposed research project or contract.

2. Pre-empting outcomes and negotiations about research
   - Members should not accept contractual conditions that are contingent upon a particular outcome or set of findings from a proposed inquiry. A conflict of obligations may also occur if the funder requires particular methods to be used.
   - Members should try to clarify, before signing the contract, that they are entitled to be able to disclose the source of their funds, its personnel, the aims of the institution, and the purposes of the project.
   - Members should also try to clarify their right to publish and spread the results of their research.
   - Members have an obligation to ensure sponsors grasp the implications of the choice between alternative research methods.

3. Guarding privileged information and negotiating problematic sponsorship
   - Members are frequently furnished with information by the funder who may legitimately require it to be kept confidential. Methods and procedures that have been utilised to produce published data should not, however, be kept confidential unless otherwise agreed.
   - When negotiating sponsorships members should be aware of the requirements of the law with respect to the ownership of and rights of access to data.
   - In some political, social and cultural contexts some sources of funding and sponsorship may be contentious. Candour and frankness about the source of funding may create problems of access or co-operation for the social researcher but concealment may have serious consequences for colleagues, the discipline and research participants. The emphasis should be on maximum openness.
   - Where sponsors and funders also act directly or indirectly as gatekeepers and control access to participants, researchers should not devolve their responsibility to protect the participants' interests onto the gatekeeper. Members should be wary of inadvertently disturbing the relationship between participants and gatekeepers since that will continue long after the researcher has left.

4. Obligations to sponsors and/or Funders During the Research Process
   - Members have a responsibility to notify the sponsor and/or funder of any proposed departure from the terms of reference of the proposed change in the nature of the contracted research.
   - A research study should not be undertaken on the basis of resources known from the start to be inadequate, whether the work is of a sociological or inter-disciplinary kind.
   - When financial support or sponsorship has been accepted, members must make every reasonable effort to complete the proposed research on schedule, including reports to the funding source.
   - Members should be prepared to take comments from sponsors or funders or research participants.
   - Members should, wherever possible, spread their research findings.
   - Members should normally avoid restrictions on their freedom to publish or otherwise broadcast research findings.

At its meeting in July 1994, the BSA Executive Committee approved a set of Rules for the Conduct of Enquiries into Complaints against BSA members under the auspices of this Statement, and also under the auspices of the BSA Guidelines on Professional Conduct. If you would like more details about the Rules, you should contact the BSA Office at the address/phone number given at the end of this statement.

British Sociological Association, Units 3F/G, Mountjoy Research Centre, Stockton Road, DURHAM, DH1 3UR [UK]. Tel.: [+44](0)191 383 0839; fax: [+44](0)191 383 0782; e-mail: *enquiries@britsoc.org.uk*

Appendix III

The Statistical Inquirer

The Statistical Inquirer is designed to assist you in learning basic statistics. There are five main activities available on the CD-R:

1   Research Files
2   Visual tutorials (video lessons on SPSS)
3   An Unsolved Mystery
4   A calculator (if you do not own one)
5   A real dataset from a study on computers and behaviour.

The answers to the lessons and to the mystery are not provided in the book or the CD–R – you will have to work them out yourself!

MINIMUM SYSTEM REQUIREMENTS

Macintosh ® PowerPC or compatible

Systems software 8.1 (or later)
20MB RAM allocated
CDROM player
256 colour monitor capable of 800×600 resolution
100MB hard disk space required

PC

Pentium class CPU
Microsoft Windows 95 (or later)
64MB system memory
CDROM player

INSTRUCTIONS

Macintosh

Double-click on the StatInquirer icon on your desk top. Transfer the StatInquirer folder to your hard disk. Open the StatInquirer folder on the hard disk and double-click on the StatInquirer icon.

The video lessons for SPSS are held on the CD–R in the Movies folder. You need to have QuickTime installed on your machine. Double click on the movie that you want to view.

PC

The CD–R should start automatically. If it does not, then go to the CD–R double click on menu.exe.

RESEARCH FILES

The research files contain library and statistics lessons. They are step-by-step lessons. If you make a mistake, then you may be given an alternative explanation or asked to key in your answer again.

Library

- finding books and articles
- databases
- Boolean operators and/or/not

Order and classification

- defining variables
- continuous and discrete variables
- arrays
- class sizes and recorded limits
- frequency distributions
- statistical tables and graphs
- general theoretical curves
- histograms and polygons
- the normal curve
- skewness

Central tendencies

- measures of central tendency
- some notation
- computing the mean for grouped data
- frequency distribution tables
- two formulae for calculating the mean of a distribution
- finding the median of a distribution
- finding the mode of a distribution

Variability

- range
- resistant measures
- mean deviation
- some notation
- Mean Absolute Deviation (MAD)
- standard deviation
- variance

Relationships

- statistical estimation
- correlation
- causation
- scatterplots
- linear relationships
- size and magnitude of relationships
- Pearson Product Moment Correlation
- regression

Statistical Inference

- samples and populations
- probability and statistical inference

DATASET

A real dataset is available on the CD–R under the file name companxi.sav. This dataset is used in the video lessons and is also available for practice in SPSS.

SPSS VIDEO LESSONS

The video lessons on SPSS are in QuickTime for Macintosh users and in Lotus ScreenCam for PC users. The lessons provide a brief introductory to:

- how to create variables in SPSS
- summary statistics
- analysing categorical variables
- one sample t-tests and chi-square
- t-tests
- regression equations
- bivariate statistics (correlations and scatterplots)
- non-parametric statistics

UNSOLVED MYSTERY

Dr Ogle has gone missing. Your task is to find out what happened to him.

Index